Entitlement Spending

Our Coming Fiscal Tsunami

Entitlement Spending

Our Coming Fiscal Tsunami

David Koitz

HOOVER INSTITUTION PRESS
Stanford University | Stanford, California

The Hoover Institution on War, Revolution and Peace, founded at Stanford University in 1919 by Herbert Hoover, who went on to become the thirty-first president of the United States, is an interdisciplinary research center for advanced study on domestic and international affairs. The views expressed in its publications are entirely those of the authors and do not necessarily reflect the views of the staff, officers, or Board of Overseers of the Hoover Institution.

www.hoover.org

Hoover Institution Press Publication No. 629

Hoover Institution at Leland Stanford Junior University,
Stanford, California, 94305-6010

First printing 2012
18 17 16 15 14 13 12   7 6 5 4 3 2 1

Manufactured in the United States of America

The paper used in this publication meets the minimum Requirements of
the American National Standard for Information Sciences—Permanence
of Paper for Printed Library Materials, ANSI/NISO Z39.48-1992. ∞

Cataloging-in-Publication Data is available from the Library of Congress
ISBN: 978-0-8179-1554-4 (cloth : alk. paper)
ISBN: 978-0-8179-1556-8 (e-book)

OUR EMERGING DILEMMA

TODAY, THE FEDERAL GOVERNMENT is facing its largest fiscal challenge since World War II.

For more than half a century, our government has routinely spent more money than it has taken in, and it has borrowed to cover its shortfalls. It has regularly rolled over its old debt into new debt, and has always made its interest payments on time. And the debt it has accumulated has been manageable. But that debt is now at its highest level in 60 years. Since 2000, it has more than tripled in dollar terms and more than doubled as a share of the economy. At the moment, the U.S. Treasury's credit rating isn't threatened. But under policies the government is now following, its future spending is projected to soar, and its need to borrow will grow precipitously.

The federal debt is now equal to almost three-fourths of the total goods and services the nation will produce this year. Within 10 years, it could approach a whole year's worth. In 25 years, it could reach two years' worth.

Despite the recent recession, the economy from which the government draws its resources is still strong and resilient. It is the world's largest, producing one-fourth of the entire world's output of goods and services. But the Treasury's outstanding debt is also accountable for one-fourth of the total debts issued by all governments worldwide.

The fundamental question before the nation is whether the government can continue on its current fiscal course. Is there a point at which its creditors will say, "Enough—your credit line has been reached"? It may seem inconceivable, but someday people may not want to buy our debt.

Many changes in taxing and spending can be implemented to overcome the threat, but at the forefront, constraints are needed on the future expenditures for Medicare, Medicaid, and Social Security. Although idolized as pillars of the nation's safety net, those programs don't stand independent of our looming fiscal problem. They are, in fact, its largest drivers. As such, if an effective remedy is to emerge, those programs must contribute heavily to the changes lawmakers consider. Simply raising taxes or borrowing more won't protect their benefits, because those actions could stifle economic growth. The ultimate "sugar daddy" for those programs is a vibrant economy. Only a healthy economy will ensure their survival because that's where the resources will come from to pay benefits to their recipients.

Debt is the worst poverty.

—Thomas Fuller (1608–1661)

CONTENTS

LIST OF FIGURES AND TABLES

Figures

Tables

PREFACE

YEARS AGO I MET with a congressman who had been serving for a long time on the Committee on Ways and Means of the U.S. House of Representatives. That committee has jurisdiction over Social Security and other entitlements, and legislation affecting those programs originates there. He was disturbed that I had been writing that the U.S. Treasury securities held by the Social Security trust funds were not real assets. As a young analyst coming to Capitol Hill in the late 1970s, I was amazed by how little members of Congress really understood about Social Security, especially about how its finances were handled. My point about the trust funds' securities was that the government does not create assets for itself when one arm issues its own securities to another arm. Those securities may have represented excess Social Security taxes collected at one time or another, but the excess money was not still sitting idly in the Treasury waiting for some future disbursement. It got used immediately to pay other government bills.

The congressman argued, "Doesn't the Treasury give the trust funds a U.S. government bond backed by the full faith and credit of the government?"

"Yes," I responded.

He went on: "And whenever those bonds have come due, hasn't the Treasury always honored them?"

Again I responded, "Yes."

"Well," he said, "what if you personally were holding a Treasury note and wanted to cash it in? Wouldn't that be an asset for you?"

"Yes," I answered.

"Okay," he said, "how can you sit there and say that the holdings of the trust funds are not real assets?"

I answered, "They are not real assets for the government. It's the right hand making promises to the left hand. What will happen," I asked, "if when the baby boomers retire, we need to draw on those promises and the government doesn't have enough taxes coming in to make good on them?"

"Look," he said, "we will simply liquidate the securities held by the trust funds and sell new securities to the public. That will give the Treasury the cash it needs. It's just a swap of one security for another."

I responded, "What that really means is the government would be writing off what it owes to itself and then borrowing what it needs. The only thing real in that transaction would be putting new bonds up for sale in the marketplace. That's borrowing, and as such, it will increase the national debt. In other words, the trust funds' holdings are simply backed by the Treasury's ability to borrow."

He answered abruptly, "So what? It's still just a swap."

For him the conversation was over.

I sat speechless. In my mind I was asking, "Since when did borrowing money become an asset for the borrower? And what happens if the day arrives when the Treasury can't borrow anymore?"

ACKNOWLEDGMENTS

I VACILLATED FOR some time before writing this monograph. As the political debate about our fiscal problems heated up in recent years, I found myself increasingly bothered by the abundance of bias and bad facts in bringing the public on board. But I had been involved with these issues on Capitol Hill for 25 years or more, and maybe I just knew too much. After all, most public policy debates are complex and value-laden, and I found myself asking if I could really add anything.

What I wanted to see was more honesty and clarity in the debate, and what finally drove me to engage was a desire for more transparency.

So I am grateful to John Cogan and John Raisian of the Hoover Institution who saw value in the direction I wanted to pursue and were willing to sponsor yet another book on this heavily—perhaps overly—trodden road of fiscal discourse. I am also grateful for two close friends, Robert Rosen and Rich McDonnell—one a Republican, the other a Democrat—who read the earliest drafts of this work, and who for years routinely engaged me with their own views as lay observers of our fiscal issues. In various ways they influenced its content, and they continue to help me shape my still-evolving understanding of the problem and the complexities of achieving a sustainable resolution.

INTRODUCTION

A FRIEND OF MINE who read an early draft of this monograph asked me why I had written it. It's already well understood on Capitol Hill that the federal government is running huge deficits and rapidly increasing its debt, and the news media have given heavy coverage to the intense machinations of the Obama Administration and lawmakers over the past few years. His comment: "The public already knows there's a big problem. What's new here?"

He's right. There's no particular illumination here of a problem buried from view. A long-unattended problem, yes. But even with that, many lawmakers acknowledge the lack of action, and the media have made much of the recent gridlock over it.

I was motivated by my perception of an abundance of filtered media and political spin that disseminate myths, misperceptions, and confusion about the problem, as reflected, for instance, by the story I relay in the preface to this book. And just as the public is coaxed to form opinions from "bad facts" and manipulative discourse, so are those directly engaged in the legislative process.

It is with this mind-set that I embarked on this project. The monograph begins with a basic narrative about the issues and their policy implications, written for a relatively easy read by the uninitiated and to be consumed in perhaps an hour or two. The appendix is a separate and distinct supplement with tables and graphs that by themselves will give the reader a simpler overview of the problem and a varied list of options to address it.

My goal was to frame a comprehensive view of the facts and, in turn, the policy direction I derive from them. I will acknowledge that I could have added more facts, perhaps other interpretations, and maybe questions regarding the reliability of future prognostications about our government's finances and the path they put us on. But to the extent there are omissions, it was in the interest of telling a cohesive story unfettered by "TMI" (too much information) and, more importantly, by an ideological or political preference.

It should be eminently obvious from the title of this book that I have my own policy bias. But there is no design here to dispute the necessity of diversity of opinion. Whatever conclusions people may want to draw, the facts about the nature and dimensions of the problem need to be transparent and broadly understood, not manufactured or otherwise colored by one's opinions.

One
OUR COMING TSUNAMI

THE UNITED STATES WILL SOON confront a major economic problem, perhaps one unparalleled in the nation's history. It won't strike tomorrow, next week, or next month, but it is out there, its roots sown by the demographics of the past half-century and a body politic hesitant to tamper with aging institutions of government. When it emerges, like a tsunami, the destructive consequences of amassing unprecedented federal indebtedness will be overwhelming, and though seemingly distant, when it rears its head it will rise suddenly in our consciousness as if coming without warning.

While a searing left-right ideological debate pervades the nation's economic dialogue, the enormity of our hovering dilemma gets short shrift. The lack of clarity in the policy discourse, the inclination by lawmakers to procrastinate on politically difficult decisions, and the propensity to pass blame and kick the can down the road are stunning. But like the tearing down of the Twin Towers, a hurricane devastating the Louisiana coast, or an earthquake striking San Francisco, our looming fiscal problem has no political division. It is not a Democratic or Republican problem. It has no party signature. It is simply an American problem. And as it draws ever closer, the need for political convergence becomes ever more pressing.

The problem is very transparent. Unlike the miasma of derivative markets or the opaque operations of hedge funds, it's not clouded by the vagaries of our financial institutions. It's a pretty straightforward dilemma. As our federal budget deficits have grown, the level of debt taken on by the U.S. Treasury has risen precipitously. Some people take solace by looking at other nations, whose debts represent a considerably larger share of their economic output, making our debt seem manageable. But given the sheer magnitude of our problem, this measure may obscure how significant even a moderate increase in the debt would be and the risk it would pose if we stay on our current course.

The challenges in our path are not modest. Starting today and continuing over the next 20 years, the post–World War II baby-boom generation will nearly double the nation's aged population, and the baby trough that followed (and has lingered since) will slow the growth of the working population. The baby boomers and the major advances in life expectancy for subsequent generations will cause a swelling number of recipients of Medicare, Medicaid, and Social Security, and the expenditures of those programs will soar, programs whose creation and inherent promises largely preceded the birth of those who now or will soon seek their benefits.

Our looming economic tsunami is simply the mountain of debt those promises portend.

Our Debt Is Not Benign

When someone asks to borrow money—which is what a country is doing when it puts its Treasury's securities up for sale—the foremost question of the lender is "If I buy these securities, what risk do I take? Is your government capable of paying me back in the period we have agreed to? Do you have a vibrant enough economy to enable your government to levy enough taxes or otherwise draw on its national resources to pay me off?"

In the growing discourse about the rising amounts of governmental debt worldwide, the common denominator of a country's creditworthiness is its debt as a percentage of what its economy produces each year. It's a proxy indicator, a way to gauge which nations are over-extended and which nations have their fiscal house under control. Eyebrows certainly get raised when a nation's debt-to-economy ratio hits triple digits. A ratio of 100 or 200 percent sets off alarms. Investors get skittish, interest rates in that country rise, and at some point, the prospect of an investor revolt ignites fears of calamity in that nation's financial markets and, potentially, those around the world.

TABLE 1.1. Debt-to-GDP Ratios for Selected Countries, Estimated 2011

Country	Percent of GDP	Country	Percent of GDP
Zimbabwe	231	United Kingdom	80
Japan	208	Israel	74
Greece	165	United States	68
Iceland	130	Spain	68
Italy	120	Netherlands	64
Ireland	107	Pakistan	60
Portugal	103	Malaysia	58
Belgium	100	Brazil	54
France	86	India	52
Canada	84	South Korea	33
Germany	82	Australia	30

Source: CIA's World Factbook, 2012.

Exactly how high does it have to go to become a concern? How much debt is too much? In 2011, Zimbabwe's debt-to-economy ratio (debt-to-GDP, or gross domestic product) was 231 percent; Japan's was 208 percent; Greece's, 165 percent; Italy's, 120 percent; Belgium's, 100 percent. Greece has certainly caught the world's attention with the fiscal turmoil it has experienced. With the possibility of default, investors got scared. Unprecedented changes in taxes and spending became necessary. Spain and Italy have also teetered on the brink, as have various other European nations. Britain too, recognizing its potentially precarious position, has undergone major belt tightening.

Can we in the U.S. take comfort because our debt-to-economy ratio was only 68 percent last year? With a lower ratio than that of other highly developed nations, with our Federal Reserve keeping short-term interest rates near zero, and with investors around the world flocking to U.S. Treasury securities as a safe haven, must we really worry? And while some countries for sure are having difficulty, other countries have markedly higher debt-to-economy ratios than we do, and they haven't collapsed or sent shock waves around the world.

For many economists, the answer is far more complicated than simply observing this ratio. What's the direction of the ratio and how rapidly is it moving (up or down)? How quickly has a high-ratio country's economy advanced and what are its future prospects? How significant are the future commitments its government has taken on? And is the country's political system stable?

The current level of U.S. Treasury debt and the direction it's headed are not benign. The U.S. may be a large and powerful nation and our debt-to-economy ratio may not be as bad as others, but that's no reason to be sanguine. Our debt will very likely go higher. The climb in our ratio from 63 percent in 2010 to 68 percent in 2011—seemingly modest—raised our Treasury debt by $1.1 trillion. That single year's rise was larger than the economies of all but 12 of the 190 nations tracked by the World Bank. It's equal to the economy of the state of New York. Absent changes that raise federal revenue or constrain spending, our debt-to-economy ratio could rise above 80 percent over the next three years, exceed 100 percent by 2024, and reach an unfathomable 200 percent by the mid-2030s.

Yes, our economy is advanced and diverse and can produce a lot. Today, it generates one-fourth of the goods and services produced worldwide. And our circumstances differ greatly from those of Greece. But when we look to the future, our governmental spending commitments are enormous. As other burgeoning countries such as China, India, South Korea, and Indonesia expand their economies, their net worth relative to ours will likely grow. Their propensity to generate larger growth rates has been demonstrated. As the Far East and South America continue their rapid spurts, how much more prominent will they become on the world's economic stage? And what happens to our dollar's strength then? As our Treasury debt continues its unrelenting rise, will the dollar and our securities still be viewed as a safe haven? Is there possibly a saturation point in the future when investors will say, "We're looking elsewhere"?

Equally important is that nearly half of our total Treasury debt is held in foreign hands, with most of that concentrated among a relatively small group of players. Three-fourths of what is owed abroad is held by China, Japan, the major oil-exporting nations, and four other countries and banking centers; 44 percent of that amount is held by China and Japan alone.[1] That makes the debt an obvious national-security concern. In early 2010, a shiver ran through the financial markets after China let go of $34 billion of our debt. The Chinese could create turmoil for us by flooding the markets with their dollar holdings, but they would also hurt themselves in the process, and that in itself serves as an impediment for exploitation. But what happens when there are other countries that become increasingly attractive for international trade and development, and our consumer demand for their goods becomes less important?

It's About Risk to Our Way of Life

Ultimately, what's at issue is our future risks: future risk to our economy, our ability to grow, our standard of living, and our national security. Today, we may be in a bubble. The dollar is king, and so are our government's securities. But where will we be in 10 years? It's not just the trajectory of our debt, but what causes it: our government's propensity to spend more than we are willing to tax ourselves. The level of debt the Treasury has issued publicly could rise to more than

---

1. Department of the Treasury, as of February 29, 2012.

$11 trillion by the end of this year, but if we count the debt it owes to the Medicare and Social Security trust funds, as well as to other "entitlement" programs—another $5 trillion—our debt-to-economy ratio suddenly rises above 100 percent.

Should we count those other obligations even though they are simply internal debt, IOUs from one arm of the government to another? Yes, because they represent future spending commitments already set in law. Lawmakers have the ability to change that, and they could raise taxes too. As yet, however, their steps have been no more than tepid, with little or no change to the fiscal path those commitments put us on. Moreover, even if we somehow came up with the money to pay off those debts (probably through more borrowing from the public), we still won't have enough coming in to pay all of the future spending commitments we've made through those programs. According to the most recent projections of the Medicare and Social Security trustees, even if those internal IOUs are paid off, the programs will run down their legal authority to spend in 2024 and 2033, respectively.[2] Taking all that into account, the Congressional Budget Office (CBO) projects that the amount of federal debt held by the public could rise to 157 percent of our annual economic production by 2032 and 200 percent by 2037. In today's dollars, it would total more than $30 trillion.

It's inconceivable that we could run up the national debt to that level. If it existed today, it would equal nearly half of what the entire world produces in a single year. Where are we going to find the

---

2. There are actually two Social Security trust funds: one for Old-Age and Survivors' Insurance and a second for Disability Insurance. The 2033 date cited in the text represents their combined point of exhaustion. Individually, the balance of the Disability Insurance trust fund is projected to fall to zero in 2016, and the Old-Age and Survivors' Insurance trust fund would fall to zero in 2035. Their combined condition is frequently used to describe the condition of the system as a whole since Congress has often reallocated the tax rates applicable to each of the two components in order to improve the status of one or the other of the two trust funds.

investors—at home or abroad—who will allow us to generate such debt? It's one thing when Zimbabwe runs up a debt of 231 percent of its economy. Its annual economic output is only $7 billion. That doesn't create economic paralyses in world markets. It's vastly different to think of the U.S. doing so. By year-end, our $11 trillion or more in publicly held debt will account for one-fourth of the $45 trillion in outstanding debt issued by all governments worldwide.[3]

As a nation, we have come to treat borrowing as simply another ready source of revenue, a spigot that we blithely presume will continually supplement what we tax ourselves. But it's not, and it won't. It's a loan that needs repaying, and as such it's a claim against future taxes—taxes that may someday fall short because the loan and our spending expectations have grown too large. There is no single trip-wire that signals danger. Complacency has a way of perpetuating itself—no pain, no worry. However, like the precipitous bursting of the tech bubble in 2000, like the air coming out of the housing market in 2008, and like investor panic over the mounting debts of established European nations, inattentiveness and procrastination toward the rising debt of the world's largest economy will someday catch up with us, likely quick and with little warning. As a policy path, the status quo won't suffice. There's no calamity at our front door today, but the warning signs are there.

It Stems from the Loss of Budgetary Control

In many ways, and through a multitude of provisions embedded in law, the federal government's spending and revenues are on autopilot. Indexing provisions tie federal revenues and spending to changes in the economy—to inflation, increases in average wages, the rise in the gross domestic product, and various other economic measures. The indexing of income-tax brackets to inflation—which keeps people's

---

3. See *The Economist,* "The Global Debt Map," 2012.

incomes from edging into higher brackets—constrains revenues. Automatic hikes of the standard deduction and personal exemptions do too. Automatic benefit increases in Social Security and other entitlement programs cause spending to rise. And benefits for Social Security recipients are automatically indexed for wage growth in the economy even before people become eligible. Automatic increases in Medicare payments to hospitals and doctors keep health-care expenditures growing at a rapid clip. The thresholds for eligibility under various anti-poverty and other support programs are automatically raised to keep needy people enrolled and allow higher benefits and reimbursements.

It's an understatement to say that indexing is embedded deeply throughout both sides of the federal ledger. In some cases it has favorable budget effects—by increasing revenues or avoiding spending—but its larger effects are to constrain revenue and increase spending.

In most if not all cases, the various indexing provisions have strong underpinnings and rationales, but they were not enacted with a larger view of the fiscal path of the nation. They were enacted incrementally, program by program, tax provision by tax provision, and in most instances with little or no overall budget plan under which to view them. It was too easy to justify them individually on programmatic or tax-policy grounds. Today, the nation's economic times are turbulent and will continue to be so over the coming decade. But those indexing provisions are still operative. They are like a faucet left running with little regard for the capacity of the well to keep delivering.

Equally instrumental is the degree of spending authorized under what are referred to as "permanent appropriations." Medicare and Social Security benefits are the primary examples. Unlike the many hundreds of programs that must receive funding approval each year through annual appropriations bills, entitlement programs such as Medicare, Medicaid, Social Security, federal and military retirement, veteran's benefits, and the like are given indefinite permission to spend through the legislation that governs them. They are on autopilot until Congress sees some reason to re-examine them, which tends to be far less frequent than with programs subjected to annual appropriation. And with the numerous programs that have indexing provisions, the autopilot nature of those provisions is facilitated by the indefinite nature of their spending authorizations.

In the nomenclature of federal budgeting, programs falling under the annual appropriations umbrella are referred to as "discretionary," as they reflect those parts of the budget where Congress routinely exercises its prerogative to raise or lower spending, to reallocate, "re-program," earmark, and even change the nature of the programs involved. The rest of the budget is comprised of "entitlements," programs that have their eligibility criteria and payments to individuals or institutions defined by the laws that created them—not by annual appropriations. These programs are labeled as "mandatory," reflecting the largely uninterrupted nature of their expenditures. Not all mandatory programs are indexed, but they do manifest the more passive role Congress takes in reviewing their goals and purposes and the multiyear (sometimes multi-decade) paths of their spending.

Mandatory spending has grown from 38 percent of the budget in 1972 to an estimated 56 percent in 2012.

FIGURE 1.1. The Portion of the Budget on "Autopilot" Now Represents More Than Half of All Federal Spending

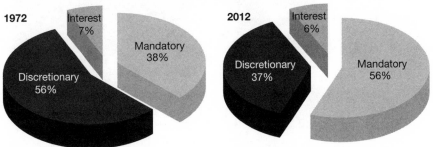

Source: Congressional Budget Office, 2012.

We Need to Change Course

Of late, the President and Congress have been focused on putting the economy back on track with stimulus measures and safety-net add-ons that increase federal spending and curtail revenues. But the public is expressing unease with the mounting budget deficits and an ever increasing national debt. Policymakers are aware of the emerging tension, and the public's unease has resulted in some resistance to enacting additional costly stimulus measures without commensurate offsets.

However, while the disquiet is palpable, so is the hesitancy. There is considerable reluctance in fiscal-policy circles to reverse the general path the federal budget is on. Among economists, the prevailing view is that tightening the fiscal belt too soon could weaken the economic recovery. For politicians, there's apprehension about the public's willingness to accept large tax increases and a retrenchment of entitlement

FIGURE 1.2. Our Twin Problems of Rising Deficits and Escalating Debt Have the Nation on an Unsustainable Fiscal Path

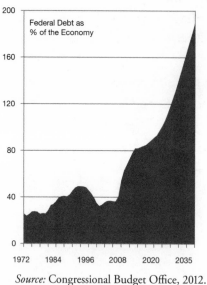
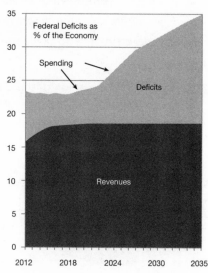

Source: Congressional Budget Office, 2012.

benefits—shorthand for raising taxes on middle- and higher-income taxpayers and constraining Medicare and Social Security benefits.

While there are those who believe the economy can grow its way out of the problem, or that painless prescriptions can be found, the more prevalent view among those who have studied the issue is that neither is really viable and neither should be relied upon. If the projections come to pass, the fear is that the fix would require sudden and severe constraints and economically stifling tax increases. Though an oversimplification, there is an old saying in the budget world: "It is better to be a pound heavy than a pound light." Politicians don't seem to have much difficulty making use of unexpected surpluses; far more stressful is finding ways to retrench if resources decline. The conventional view among fiscal-policy watchers is that the earlier we adopt serious change, the smaller it needs to be. That window, however, grows shorter every year—especially now that the baby-boom retirees are already coming on to the Medicare and Social Security rolls.

So Where Do We Look?

As goes the old fable about the bank robber Willie Sutton—a reporter asks, "Willie, why do you rob banks?" and he answers, "Because that's where the money is"—any effort to rein in our budget deficits and the Treasury debt they leave us with will mean homing in on where the money is. The quandary is that recent opinion polls indicate the public doesn't really understand where it is.

Many want to blame the deficits on too many wasteful programs: extravagant earmarks, bridges to nowhere, defective weapons system, fraud in Medicare and Medicaid, non-competitive contracting, pork-barrel politicking, and congressional perks. All those targets may be valid examples of excess, but on the whole, they impart a narrow prescription. They suggest that the hole can be plugged by weaning out "bad" spending.

The difficulty is that one man's waste is often another man's honest production. The chorus is loud: "Federal spending on schools is excessive, but my school district needs more money." "That bridge did not need to be built in your state, but the highways in my state are full of potholes." "We spend too much on defense, but don't shut down that jet-engine plant across town." The chorus feeds on the premise "just cut the fat; no need to slice the muscle." The problem comes in distinguishing between the two.

Discretionary spending is the one area where Congress exercises considerable choice. In the aggregate, this area involves substantial expenditures that now constitute 37 percent of the budget. And it is the part of the budget where the public perceives an abundance of excess and wasteful earmarks. But discretionary spending is not a hodgepodge of overspending. Disclosures of waste by the military notwithstanding, having effective armed forces is costly. And while spending on defense and the two wars has been quite large, even at its current elevated levels it is only 18 percent of the budget this year. Welfare programs are only 10 percent of the budget;[4] education spending is 2 percent; the National Institutes of Health (NIH), 1 percent; farm programs, less than 1 percent; the national parks and conservation programs, the same.

True, there are a multitude of discretionary programs to explore for savings, but as many budget hawks have observed, it's hard to take them on en masse given the multitude of special interests that rise up in arms. Every lawmaker's district has something to protect. The fight for the small savings is almost as hard as that for major ones. And as the title of this component of the budget implies, discretion imparts the ability to choose, meaning lawmakers can raise spending as readily as cut it.

---

4. Other than Medicaid. Consists mostly of cash assistance and related spending, e.g., food stamps and housing assistance.

The debate may be contentious, but the math is overwhelming: the big money lies with Medicare, Medicaid, and Social Security benefits. Nearly 50 million people now have Medicare coverage, some 70 million are enrolled in Medicaid at various times during the year, and 57 million people get Social Security benefits. Those numbers will only swell as the baby boomers continue to enter their senior years. Those big three entitlements are the major drivers of the long-range escalation of government spending.

FIGURE 1.3. The Big Three Entitlements Are the Major Drivers of Future Federal Spending

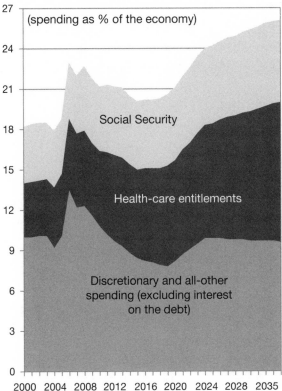

Source: Congressional Budget Office, 2012.

Notably, federal taxes as a share of the economy now sit close to their lowest level in 60 years—15.7 percent in 2012. Since the early 1950s, taxes on average have absorbed about 18 percent of the economy. But even if they were to rise to this historical average, they would be no match for the dramatic increase in federal spending over the next two decades driven by the big three entitlements and growing interest on the debt.

Whatever the prescription for change, policies that raise large amounts of revenue or significantly constrain spending—balanced or not—are assuredly contentious. Raise taxes and the Chamber of Commerce and National Federation of Independent Business talk about economic stagnation. Attack farm subsidies and farm-state politicians raise their shields. Mention Medicare and Social Security cuts and AARP and the vast network of social-welfare advocates erupt. The anti-tax crowd raises the tax-and-spend argument. The protect-entitlements crowd argues it's a conspiracy by conservatives to undo the safety net. The arguments get twisted, the facts get lost: "We can grow our way out of it." "Just get rid of the waste." "Stop illegal immigrants from draining our welfare system." "Raise taxes on the rich." "Increased spending will grow the economy." "Larger business tax preferences will do the same."

All sides can make a case. Individually, they may be defensible. Where they lose merit is when put in the context of the greater economy. The fact is we as a nation want our taxes to be low and our entitlements to be comprehensive. And if that means more borrowing, so be it. For many years that worked, but the clock is ticking now toward a problematic climax. There will be a day of reckoning with the debt we're accumulating. The old defenses won't work because it will be the financial markets that drive us. Angry Social Security recipients won't budge bond buyers who won't buy our Treasury securities. Politicians can't pass laws to make them lend us money. The Federal Reserve can do only so much for so long to quell rising interest rates. Enacting usury laws won't open the wallets of foreign investors.

A nation deep in debt is no different from an individual or family that is over-extended. And the solutions are the same: raise household income or curtail spending.

Our Critical Juncture Is Now

Beyond the risks that drive the need to restore fiscal discipline, there is the larger question of what rising entitlement spending implies about our aging society. The nation is at a critical juncture with our economic policies. Our economic well-being does not rest on protecting the amount of government spending people receive or on keeping their tax burden light. It rests on the continued vibrancy of our economy. While protecting safety-net programs and repelling higher taxes may appear to be standing up for the masses, when doing so threatens the economy it threatens the masses.

TABLE 1.2. The Aged Share of the Population Will Rise From One-in-Eight to One-in-Five in Twenty Years

Year	Total Population	Number Who Are 65 or Older	Aged Population as Share of Total Population
	(millions of people)		(percent)
2012	320	43	13
2025	357	65	18
2035	381	78	20
2050	409	84	20

Source: Social Security trustees' report, 2012.

With the baby boomers now entering their retirement years and longevity continuing to rise, the Medicare and Social Security trustees estimate that in little more than a decade the number of people aged 65 and older will increase from 43 million to 65 million—more than a 50 percent rise by 2025. Where they make up 13 percent of the total population today, they will grow to 18 percent in 2025. By 2035, their numbers will reach 78 million, and they will be 20 percent of the population.

As the population ages, one of the major engines of economic growth—an expanding workforce—will slow substantially due to the large exodus of older workers from the labor force and the lower birth rates following the post–World War II baby boom. This combination of factors presents a distinct challenge for the economy, which will be called upon to devote a large and rising share of what it produces to retirees.

The significance of this shift is reflected by the decline in the number of workers per aged person that is projected to occur by 2030. In 1970, there were 4.4 workers for every aged person. Over the subsequent 30 years, the growth in the number of workers was more than four times that of the aged population, keeping the ratio of workers to aged persons relatively constant. In contrast, the Medicare and Social Security actuaries project that from 2020 to 2030 the reverse

TABLE 1.3. The Number of Workers for Every Retiree Is Starting a Long-Term Decline

Year	Increase in workers during previous decade	Increase in population aged 65+ during previous decade	Ratio of workers to population aged 65+
	(millions of people)		
1970	20.5	3.6	4.4
1980	19.7	5.3	4.3
1990	20.4	5.7	4.2
2000	21.5	3.8	4.3
2010	2.4	5.4	3.8
2020	16.7	14.6	3.1
2030	7.5	17.1	2.5

Source: Social Security trustees' report, 2012.

will occur: the increase in the aged population will more than double that of the working population, and by 2030, there will be only 2.5 workers for every aged person.

Food, clothing, medical care, and the many other services needed by the aged cannot be stored in advance. Thus, to a large extent the goods and services that society will consume will have to be produced then. Because of the slowly growing labor force, however, the economy is not expected to expand as rapidly as it has over the last half-century.

Projections of Medicare and Social Security costs for the next 20 years reflect those pressures. As a share of GDP, Medicare's expenditures are projected to rise from 3.7 percent this year to 6.0 percent in 2032; Social Security's would rise from 5.0 percent to 6.1 percent. While both are seemingly small, that's an increase of more than 60 percent for Medicare and 22 percent for Social Security. As a share of today's GDP, it would be equivalent to a $530 billion increase in federal spending this year—nearly a one-sixth rise. Moreover, the demographic trend emerging with the baby boomers' retirement is not a temporary bulge in the proportion of elderly to non-elderly but a long-term shift to an older society caused by increasing longevity and persistently low birth rates. And because other sources of retirement benefits—pensions and other health-care programs—will also be affected, projections of Medicare and Social Security spending portray only a portion of the total costs of retirees for society.

It has been suggested that if birth rates remain low, the rising costs of the aged might be offset by the lower costs of raising fewer children—the implication being that the overall dependency on workers may not be all that troublesome. Current actuarial projections show that the number of people who are not of primary working age—people under 20 and those 65 or older—won't make up any higher a percentage of the population than they did when the baby boomers were in their youth.

But that comparable ratio of dependents to workers does not mean that America's aging will impose little burden on tomorrow's workers.

That ratio obscures the much greater cost of supporting each senior. Studies have shown that governmental income support and health-care spending for the aged (by all levels of government) substantially exceed governmental spending associated with educating and providing services to children. As the percentage of the population that is elderly goes up, pressures will build on public budgets to a much greater extent than at any time since World War II. Moreover, the level of dependency on working-age adults is not projected to fall when the baby boomers die, as it did when they emerged from childhood.

Finally, aside from the cost disparity, there is a profound societal difference between sacrificing to build for the future—as we do when we spend on children—and sacrificing to subsidize the living standard of the elderly. Both may be regarded as desirable social goals, but the former is largely an investment that bears returns over time while the latter is largely consumption. Thus, the shifting demographics we now face portend a spending burden that is both higher and more consumption-oriented than we experienced during the baby boomers' youth.

If the nation is to meet the rising demand for goods and services, it must invest more to spur productivity so that the greater demand can be met by fewer people. Finding the resources to meet that demand will be much easier in a growing economy than in a stagnant one, and the best way to achieve that result is to increase national saving. Increasing national saving will provide the capital to finance investments, which in turn will increase the amount of goods and services each worker can produce.

If lawmakers simply schedule future tax increases to pay for future consumption, it will mean little if the economy has not expanded sufficiently. It would amount to a zero-sum game in which any gain for Medicare and Social Security recipients would come at the expense of the rest of the budget, the economy, and future generations of workers. Doing that is little more than procrastinating about the issue, and procrastinating about taking hard steps today amounts to a gamble that future lawmakers will make the necessary decisions to cut consumption or just succumb to a potentially stagnating or degenerative economy. Any way you look at it, that's passing the buck.

Businesses and individuals can do two things with their money: they can use it to buy things, or they can save it. To nurture a growing economy, we need to save. When people and institutions save, they supply the capital to finance investments that enhance productivity. The same is true when making government policy. There are many possible tracks the government could take to increase saving, but there is a pretty strong consensus that the most direct way is to rein in government borrowing that saps investment resources from the financial markets. That means reducing budget deficits (or, however implausible it seems today, running budget surpluses). And that requires raising taxes or constraining spending. Simply put, there is no hedging in achieving national saving.

Ideological factors often confound the debate, but the fundamental question is "What is most likely to result in genuine saving?" Which legal, political, and fiscal incentives best ensure that resources are actually reallocated from the present to the future? While raising taxes to reduce government borrowing might appear equal to constraining spending, the magnitude of the tax hikes needed to match the rising expenditures could very well impede business investment, personal saving, and work effort. Constraining government expenditures that add to consumption, adopting policies that advance productive technology and investment in education, eliminating government regulations that inhibit productivity, and adopting tax measures that reward personal saving and work are the types of policies likely to have the greatest chance of spurring growth.

For many, constraining government consumption—entitlement expenditures—may seem counterintuitive. How can future retirees be better off if their benefits have been constrained? The answer is that if the economy grows larger as a consequence of those decisions, the benefits paid in the future may retain or even increase their value. For instance, Social Security benefits that absorb 4 percent of an economy that has doubled may be richer than those absorbing 6 percent of an economy that has seen only modest expansion.

Even if not culminating in a financial meltdown, the projected rise in entitlement spending, left unabated, would weigh heavily on the economy as an ever rising share of workers' earnings and business profits are siphoned off to pay for these programs. If not that, much of the capital available for investment will go elsewhere in the world or be soaked up by a massive public debt. Medicare costs will create the most strain, followed closely by Social Security and Medicaid, and together they will have the potential to devour our productive capacity. Slowing their long-term growth would help prevent escalating debt, ease the pressure for much higher taxes, and leave more resources available in the financial markets for investment.[5]

Pragmatism Must Override Social Dogma

While perceived as pillars of the nation's safety net, Medicare and Social Security serve a much broader population than the poor and disabled, and their expenditures for the middle class and higher-income population are vastly greater than those for poor and near-poor recipients. Characterized as a form of insurance—social insurance—they serve virtually the entire workforce and their families, the idea being that all workers need to have a stake in the programs for them to address the

---

5. The preceding section builds off of discussions of the broad economic impact of society's aging in earlier pieces by the author published by the Congressional Budget Office and the Concord Coalition. See *Long-Range Fiscal Policy Brief No. 8,* "Acquiring Financial Assets to Fund Future Entitlements," Congressional Budget Office, June 16, 2003, and "Social Security Series: A Real Fix for Social Security Requires an Increase in National Savings," Concord Coalition, April 13, 2005.

broad range of risks people face over their lifetimes. Lessening those risks on society is the principle on which they rest.

For decades that principle has served as a powerful bulwark against those who would challenge their existence. To limit or curtail social-insurance benefits for people of moderate or above-average means was heresy—the logic being that limiting or curtailing their benefits would be tantamount to means testing, and means testing would turn Medicare and Social Security into programs for the poor alone. To recite the conventional dogma, "a program for the poor will always be a poor program."

Standing on principle is admirable, and there is much truth to be found in our experience with welfare programs (welfare is not popular, and with some exception, its funding is routinely challenged). But when push comes to shove and the safety net starts threatening the very economic base from which its resources derive, dogma can be counterproductive. A program for the poor may be a poor program, but when a program for the masses threatens the economy, it can make for a poor economy.

More to the point, the motivation for trimming government entitlements involves more than an ideological challenge from the right or a theoretical question of whether it will turn a program into welfare. It's as much about the need to save money. It's about where the money will come from to pay for our bulging entitlement programs and everything else we want from the economy.

When push comes to shove, we will need to tighten our belt, and as the wealthiest nation on earth, we have the ability to do so while protecting the poor and disabled. The politics of retrenchment are hardly inviting. The difficulty is obvious: to the extent it hits the middle class, it causes heartburn for politicians of both parties. But holding to the premise that the only way to protect society against the economic perils of life is by having the government spend hundreds of billions of dollars every year on rich and poor alike is false savings. Somewhere along the way, we, as a generation fortunate enough to be living in the most prosperous of times, have lost sight of a very basic tenet, and that is you cannot have what you cannot afford or do not want to pay for. Social insurance cannot be unbounded. With the path we are on, we are biting the hand that feeds us—our economy. And by impeding the future economy with enormous debt or large tax increases, everyone will suffer.

Two
FACING UP TO THE ELEPHANTS IN THE ROOM:
Medicare and Medicaid

WITH SPENDING ON HEALTH CARE in the United States accounting for one out of six dollars of the nation's annual economic output,
the amount of national income devoted to maintaining our health
status affects our economic well-being and the way we live. Having
grown more than three-fold as a share of the economy over the past
half-century, the nation's health-care system now suffers from a host
of entrenched problems. It's too complicated, provides uneven care,
leaves too many people without insurance, is over-burdened with a
maze of claims-making rules and bureaucracy, and is inordinately
costly. On a per capita basis we have the most expensive system in
the world. Consuming nearly $8,000 per person in 2009, our health-
care costs were more than twice as high as the average of other major
developed countries. But as routinely exhibited by broad measures of
well-being, our health status lags behind.

Like other nations, we've enjoyed considerable gains in life expectancy over the past half-century, but we are still back in the pack.
Measured from birth, our life expectancy rose more than eight years
between 1960 and 2009. In Japan the increase was more than 15 years,
and the average in all OECD countries was more than 11 years. Our

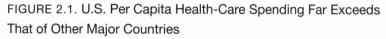

FIGURE 2.1. U.S. Per Capita Health-Care Spending Far Exceeds
That of Other Major Countries

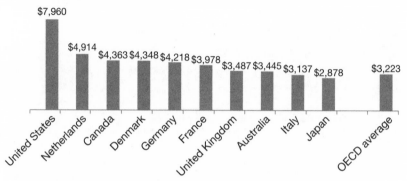

Source: Organization for Economic Cooperation and Development (OECD), 2012;
figures for 2009.

infant mortality rates have improved as well, standing at 6.5 deaths
per 1,000 live births in 2008, but the OECD average was 4.4 in 2009.
In Iceland, Sweden, Finland, and Japan the rates were around 2.5.
In contrast to those measures of improved health, obesity rates have
worsened across many countries, and here too we have lagged. Our
obesity rate among adults was 33.8 percent in 2008. Among 14 other
countries where obesity could be measured, the average was 21 percent. Obesity is a precursor to various health problems, in particular
diabetes and cardiovascular disease, and its growing prevalence serves
as a strong indicator of even higher health-care costs in the future.[1]

The Intractable Problem: The Rising Price of Medical Care

National health expenditures in the U.S., public and private combined, are projected to reach $2.8 trillion this year. In 1960, at $27
billion, they represented 5 percent of what the economy produced

---

1. See OECD Health Data 2011 for the United States, "How Does the United States
Compare."

FIGURE 2.2. National Spending for Health Care Has Grown Rapidly as a Share of the Economy.

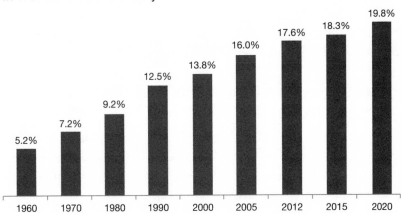

Source: Centers for Medicare & Medicaid Services, 2012.

and spent. Over the following 50 years, they routinely outpaced the growth of the economy, and could reach 17.6 percent this year and 20 percent by 2020.[2]

For more than half a century health-care prices have risen with a heavy dose of impunity, far outstripping inflation and the rise in workers' incomes. And the implications of that growth now extend well beyond traditional health-care concerns, making it perhaps the major factor in finding a sustainable direction for national economic policy.

Rapidly rising health-care prices are the deep-rooted cancer in our economic system. Growing with little restraint, they make health insurance expensive, make employers reluctant to provide coverage, dissuade people from buying insurance, keep ill people from seeking timely medical care, make our business sector less competitive in world markets, absorb an inordinate amount of our personal income,

---

2. See Centers for Medicare & Medicaid Services, "National Health Expenditures, 2012"—historical and projected series.

take money away from other public priorities, and help drive up the public debt.

Perhaps nowhere is the conundrum more evident and more disturbing than in the financial state of the two largest sources for paying the population's health-care bills: Medicare and Medicaid.

TABLE 2.1. Growth of Medicare and Medicaid as Payers of Medical Care*

Year	Medicare spending	Medicaid spending	Total national spending on medical care	Medicare and Medicaid's share of the nation's total spending on medical care
	($ billions)			
1970	7.7	5.3	67.1	19.4%
1980	37.4	26.0	235.7	26.9%
1990	110.3	73.7	675.6	27.2%
2000	224.3	200.5	1,289.6	32.9%
2012	565.6	456.8	2,646.9	38.6%

*Note: Table reflects spending for "personal health care," which is a subset of national health expenditures.
Source: Centers for Medicare & Medicaid Services, National Health Expenditures, 2012.

The economic stress affecting Medicare and Medicaid is immediate, and has been steadily intensifying for years. Medicare, the nation's largest single source of health-care funding, now spends much more than the taxes and premiums it brings into the Treasury—$275 billion more last year. In fact, for most of its history, Medicare spending has exceeded its revenues, and on average, people today receive far more in benefits than they paid in taxes and premiums.[3] Medicaid, the nation's second-largest source of health-care funding, has grown 18-fold since

---

3. See, for instance, "Social Security and Medicare Taxes and Benefits Over a Lifetime," by C. Eugene Steuerle and Stephanie Rennane, Urban Institute, June 20, 2011.

1980 and now provides health benefits for nearly 70 million people, or almost a quarter of the total population. With its costs shared with the federal government, Medicaid expenditures exceed one-fifth of overall spending by state governments and have been straining the budgets of most states for years.[4] In 2011, annual federal spending for both Medicare and Medicaid ($850 billion) exceeded spending on Social Security ($727 billion) and national defense ($700 billion) and represented almost a quarter of the Treasury's total budget outlays.

TABLE 2.2. Changes in Average Annual Per Capita Medical-Care Spending, 1969–2010

Year	Under Medicare	Under private health insurance
	(percent)	
1969–1993	10.9	12.8
1993–1997	7.2	4.3
1997–1999	−0.5	6.2
1999–2002	6.3	8.6
2002–2007	7.9	6.7
1969–2010	8.7	10.0

Source: Centers for Medicare & Medicaid Services, National Health Expenditures, 2012.

Medicare is entirely managed and funded by the federal government, and financed primarily by taxes paid by workers and their employers and premiums paid by people enrolled in the program.

4. Includes the federal share of Medicaid funding. Actual Medicaid spending from state general funds hovers around 17 percent. Education remains the largest use of state funds, but state Medicaid spending, counting both federal and state funding shares, closely matches spending on education. Overall, in recent decades, state Medicaid spending has been growing considerably faster than state spending on education and all other major components of state budgets.

Medicaid is funded by both the federal and state governments and operated by the states, serving primarily the lowest-income segments of the population. The medical care funded by the two programs is mostly provided through the non-governmental sector, and the payment rates for services are set by the respective governments.

Periodically, the federal government or a state have attempted to constrain one form of payment or another, whether it be to hospitals or physicians, but in due course political pressures caused the programs to adjust such that their spending generally tracks with that of other health-care insurers. For example, from 1969 to 2010, like national health expenditures in the aggregate, per-enrollee spending under Medicare far outstripped the growth in the economy, but at a somewhat slower rate than that of private health insurance. Since the early 1990s, however, spending by governmental health programs in the aggregate has been growing more rapidly than private spending, largely due to expansions in coverage.[5]

While provider reimbursements under Medicare and Medicaid are based on health-care prices generally, it's uncertain exactly how spending under the two programs affects the national trajectory of health-care costs. Clearly, the programs do not function in isolation. They fund health care by using the nation's vast network of providers: hospitals, doctors, nursing homes, home-health agencies, educational facilities, and so on. And as the nation's largest payers of medical bills—financing more than one-third of all medical care—they are the elephants in the room. Since their arrival 47 years ago, they have substantially increased demand for health care and stimulated supply.

Which has been the more dominant effect can only be conjectured. Some would suggest that, whatever their effects on supply and demand,

---

5. Examples of expansion of coverage include enactment of prescription-drug coverage under Medicare and the State Children's Health Insurance Program (SCHIP).

much of the higher prices is due to technological advancements, new medicines, and new treatments. Others contend that, as third-party payers, the two programs have come between the consumer of service and the provider, and have helped erode consumers' sensitivity to the price of medical care.

To which extent either of those has been the dominant driver is similarly conjecture. Most likely, one feeds on the other as third-party financing reduces incentives for the doctor or patient to question the efficacy of innovations. But what isn't conjecture is that Medicare and Medicaid, through their amalgamation with the nation's suppliers of medical services, contribute to and are affected by the rapid rise in our spending on health care.

FIGURE 2.3. Medicare and Medicaid's Share of Paying for the Nation's Health Care Has Doubled over the Past 40 Years

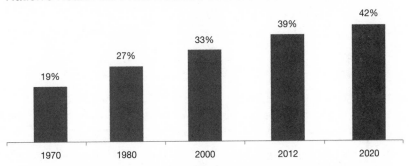

Source: Centers for Medicare & Medicaid Services, 2012.

Both CBO and Medicare's trustees assume some long-range savings from President Obama's sponsored 2010 health-care law (the Affordable Care Act), but Medicare's upward cost trajectory is only modestly constrained. Under those projections, as a share of the economy, the program would still double in size over the next 25 years. Taken together with new federal subsidies to help uninsured people buy health insurance and other mandatory spending on health care—

particularly an increase in the federal government's share of Medicaid—federal spending on health-care entitlements is projected to rise from 5.4 percent of the nation's GDP in 2012 to 10.4 percent in 2037.[6] If spending at that level were to prevail today, it would represent half of the entire federal budget (excluding interest on the debt), and by itself would account for more than 10 cents out of every dollar of the nation's annual production of goods and services.

TABLE 2.3. Medicare and Medicaid's Growing Share of Federal Primary Spending (i.e., Everything but Interest on the Debt)

Year	Medicare and Medicaid	Social Security	All other primary spending
	(percent of the economy)		
2012	5.4	5.0	11.6
2015	6.4	5.1	9.7
2025	7.9	5.7	9.1
2037	10.4	6.2	9.6

Source: Congressional Budget Office, "The Long-Term Budget Outlook," 2012.

Some will argue that the projections are wrong, that they are too pessimistic, that they don't reflect the real "savings" potential under a variety provisions in the 2010 legislation, or that the economy will become much more robust as the recovery from the recent recession advances. There are lots of what-ifs to attack the outlooks, but the

---

6. See CBO's alternative fiscal scenario in its report on the "Long-Term Budget Outlook," 2012. This alternative scenario to the agency's current law forecast (often referred to as the baseline forecast) represents a future budget path that assumes little change in recent fiscal policies: i.e., from what might be viewed as the status quo. Under CBO's projections, national spending on health, which stood at just under 10 percent of GDP in 1985, is assumed to rise from 17 percent of GDP in 2010 to 25 percent in 2037.

principal factors that underpin them are deeply seeded. The first is our "aging" demographics; the second, our long history of rapid health-care inflation. Those are not flash-in-the-pan phenomena—baby boomers are becoming senior boomers and our society is aging now. And health-care prices have outstripped the growth of the economy for decades. True, the future is always uncertain, but to dismiss those potential drivers of health-care spending is myopic. With what's in front of us, one could just as readily conclude the assumptions aren't pessimistic enough.

Over the next two decades, the aged—the largest per capita consumers of health care[7]—are projected to grow sharply as a share of the population. For much of the past 50 years, they comprised about one in 10 people in the population. Over the next 10 years, that number is projected to rise to nearly one in six. Over the next 20 years, it could reach one in five.

The analogy is often made that the retirement of the baby boomers is like a pig being swallowed by a python. But the analogy hardly tells the story. Yes, there is a swelling about to emerge, but no contraction is projected to follow when the baby boomers eventually die off. The nation's population has been aging steadily because of improvements in life expectancy and a slowing birth rate. In effect, with the baby boomers' entrance into their advanced years, there is now emerging a permanent step-up to a population comprised of many more older people and, with it, a society with a much greater propensity to consume health care.

---

7. In this regard, it should be observed that from 1987 to 2004 persons 65 and older represented 12 percent of the total population, but accounted for roughly 35 percent of the nation's total spending for personal health care. *Source:* Centers for Medicare & Medicaid Services, Office of the Actuary, National Health Statistics Group.

TABLE 2.4. Personal Health-Care Spending
by Age, 2004

Spending per capita for population:		
Age 65+	Working age	Children
$14,797	$4,511	$2,650

Source: U.S. Health Spending by Age, Selected Years
Through 2004, *Health Affairs,* November 2007.

The rapid rise in federal health-care spending is the largest potential driver of the federal government's long-range budget spending.
The aggregate expenditures of Medicare and Medicaid, propelled
by the rapid rise in health-care costs, will only be amplified by the
emerging population trends. The oldest baby boomers, born in 1946,
became eligible for Medicare last year. Over the next 20 years, their
generation will swamp Medicare and Medicaid. One needs only to
recognize that population shift to understand the enormous struggle
lawmakers will shortly confront over the shrinking availability of federal resources. Today, Medicare's revenues are paying for only 60 percent of its benefits, and the program is increasingly relying on the
government's general receipts, including those obtained from borrowing. Certainly, everything we label as discretionary—defense spending, education assistance, road and bridge construction, agricultural
support, NIH research, environmental programs, public assistance,
housing, airports and airways, etc.—will be threatened.

Confounding as it may be for funding other federal programs,
this dramatic increase in health-care spending will weigh heavily on
the economy. Whether through excessive government borrowing or
higher taxes, an ever rising share of the nation's available investment
capital would be diverted to maintain a grossly inefficient national
system of health care whose costs are out of control.

The Administration's recent efforts to extend health insurance to
the uninsured and lessen the insurance inefficiencies that deny coverage

serve the noble goal of trying to better meet the nation's health-care needs. But we are not entering a period conducive to spending more public dollars to get those results. Our problem with publicly financed health care is much greater than figuring out how the government can pay for new benefits. The stress of paying for what we have now has already reached a critical stage. With the aggregate projected rise in federal spending and slower revenue growth, the large budget deficits we see today will pale in comparison to those that could emerge in the future.

Politicians are generally reluctant to talk about the hard medicine of reform, but in failing to do so they fail to educate the public that we are at the end of the period when we can afford unrestrained entitlements.[8]

---

8. For further discussion, also see "The Nation's Health Care Conundrum: Where Do We Go From Here?," by David Koitz, Concord Coalition, May 15, 2009.

Three

CUTTING THROUGH THE SOCIAL SECURITY FOG

LAST YEAR, 158 MILLION of us paid Social Security taxes, and in return for continuing to do so, most of us will receive Social Security someday. Some 57 million of us already do, and nearly 6 million more will join the rolls this year. Since its inception, more than 230 million people have been awarded benefits. Whether you are now aged 23 or 67, you are probably in the Social Security pool in some way, and you probably have some opinion about how Social Security works—whether it's fair or unfair, whether it takes too much out of your pay, whether it will or will not be there when it's your turn, whether you could have done better with your money. Start a conversation about Social Security and everyone will have something to say.

The problem is so few of us really understand it—even the basics.

It starts with the esoteric. The Social Security Act has 21 titles, of which the program we call Social Security is only one. It has 34 sections, hundreds of sub-sections, and thousands of sub-sub-sections, not to mention the many other laws that have a Social Security component. All told, the compilation of Social Security and related laws exceeds 2,000 pages, reflecting thousands of amendments enacted since the original act was passed in 1935. And not to start a debate about whether it is Social Security or the federal tax code that is most arcane, but Social Security would at least run a close second.

When I ran a policy shop on the Hill and mentored new staff, my monotonous, persistent admonition was "keep it simple." Entitlement programs in general are swamped with minute details and complexity. Members of Congress, being a reflection of the public, are more likely to form a perception of how these programs work from some 30-second segment on the nightly news than from some grounded understanding of them. With its voluminous coffer of jargon and technical language, Social Security has the propensity to baffle even the most initiated lawmaker. So much so that one could easily conclude that understanding Social Security is an oxymoron.

But even putting that density aside, what is simple is often made complex and confusing by proponents and antagonists of the program who take advantage of jargon and technical imagery to drive a point of view. It's the battle to influence public perception that often obscures fact from fiction. And perhaps nothing has confused the public more than the debate about where Social Security taxes go and how Social Security affects the federal budget and the government's emerging fiscal problem.

The basics are simple:

- Social Security is a federal program;
- Its taxes are federal taxes;
- Those taxes and the benefits paid to its recipients flow into and out of the federal Treasury;
- And, as with all other programs of the government, the Treasury Department keeps track of those transactions through separate accounts.

The jargon is not so simple:

- There are terms like "insurance," as in the legal title of the program, "Old-Age, Survivors, and Disability Insurance";

- Recipients are referred to as "beneficiaries" and benefits as "primary insurance amounts";
- Taxes are labeled "contributions," as in "the Federal Insurance Contributions Act" and "the Self-Employment Contribution Act," or FICA and SECA;
- Record keeping by the Treasury is done through "trust funds." There are two, one for Old-Age and Survivors' Insurance and the other for Disability Insurance;
- And excess income is deemed to be an "investment."

Most formidable are the technical concepts delineating the program's financial condition and the evaluations of whether its future income will be sufficient to meet its future spending.

The program's trust-fund accounts hold U.S. Treasury securities that have maturity dates and earn interest. Open the annual Social Security trustees' report and there is a whole page listing the federal bonds, federal notes, and federal certificates of indebtedness that make up the balances of the trust funds and represent the accumulation of excess taxes and other "income" recorded by the Treasury to the funds. They are legal forms of government indebtedness, but in reality they are merely "paper" credits from one arm of the government to another. Their purpose is to give the Treasury Department permission to spend, meaning that as long as the trust funds have a balance posted to them, the secretary of the Treasury is authorized to pay benefits. Beyond that, there is no real economic value to them.

To accentuate the distinction, unlike the securities the Treasury issues at public auctions, the trust funds' securities are non-marketable—truly another oxymoron if one dwells on it. They have no commercial value, as they cannot be bought, sold, or traded in the financial markets. They are basically a form of internal record keeping, institutionalized to "authorize" Social Security payments from the Treasury. They represent a "lid" of sorts on what can be spent, but they have no true value in the context that most laypeople would think of an asset.[1]

Not to disparage those who believe that there once was a separate pot of Social Security money that had real value, but the truth is there is no such entity and never has been. There isn't a Fidelity Investments or T. Rowe Price money-market fund or investment portfolio, or any other managed fund of stocks and bonds, to be used exclusively for Social Security purposes. It's the U.S. Treasury that finances the system. What people pay and receive under the umbrella of Social Security is a Treasury transaction, and it has been that way since taxes were first levied for the program in 1937.

If there is a perception of chicanery, it likely stems from the view that Social Security as an "institution" has been exploited to serve purposes other than what people believe was intended—that somehow its original design of providing retirement annuities was diluted. As the argument goes, "If Congress raised benefits, they weakened the trust funds' reserves. If they made more people eligible for benefits, they raided their assets." The fact is that when Congress passed legislation liberalizing Social Security over the years—regardless of whether lawmakers raised commensurate revenue—the money always flowed into and out of the Treasury, not the trust funds, and there was no build up of what one would consider hard or tangible assets to pay those benefits.

The term "trust fund" is a mere label. Every program of the government has a Treasury account to track its finances, and many of the

---

1. The non-marketable distinction here should not be overemphasized. It helps make the point that the holdings of the trust funds do not represent assets for the government in any conventional sense. However, even if the trust funds held marketable federal securities, they would have no intrinsic value for the government. They would still represent one arm of the government making a promise—an IOU—to another arm of the government. And selling them to the public would still represent borrowing in the same form as the Treasury issuing new federal securities for sale to finance any other function of government.

largest, like Social Security, have the distinction of being labeled a trust fund. That label doesn't mean that something different is done with Social Security monies or those of other "trust fund" programs. It all flows to and from the Treasury.

Social Security Is Very Much a Contributor to the Government's Fiscal Outlook

If one follows the conventional portrayal of Social Security's finances in its annual trustees' reports, the problem garnering the greatest attention is "When will the trust funds become exhausted—when will their balances fall to zero?" Certainly that's what the media homes in on. According to the 2012 trustees' report, the trust funds would not run out until 2033.[2] And presumably it is from that point on that the program would have insufficient income to fully cover the benefits that are scheduled under the benefit rules in current law.

That would be the technical, legal view of the program's insolvency, as 2033 would be the point at which the Secretary of the Treasury's "reserve" spending authority would be exhausted, and he would be forced to suspend or reduce the benefits otherwise required.

That, however, is a narrow view of Social Security's troubles. The real problem is not distant. It's not 21 years away. It's here today as part of the larger problem caused by 60 years of deficit spending by the federal government and especially the extraordinary run-up of federal debt over the past decade. For years, the argument in defense of Social Security has been that the system carries its own weight and has raised more taxes than it has spent. And the frequent rejoinder to including Social Security in any search for budget savings has been "Social Security is not the problem, it's everything else."

---

2. See "The 2012 Annual Report of the Board of Trustees of the Federal Old-Age and Survivors Insurance and Federal Disability Insurance Trust Funds," Washington, D.C., April 25, 2012.

Though a naive perspective of how federal tax policy has been made, that view has been deeply implanted in public discourse and perception. In the real world, Social Security has not evolved as an entity separate and distinct from other functions of the government and the fiscal decisions made by lawmakers. When its taxes were levied and periodically raised, they became part of the overall federal tax burden that workers and their employers must carry. And for much of the past half-century, Social Security taxes have been the largest of all those paid by most workers—federal, state, or local. While income taxes and other forms of federal taxation may not have been significant enough to keep the federal budget balanced, they were not set in ignorance of how large Social Security taxes were for workers and their employers.

It's a pretty dubious argument to suggest that members of Congress's tax-writing committees were not conscious of the burden of Social Security taxes when setting federal income-tax rates. Enactment of the Earned Income Tax Credit in the early 1970s was heavily motivated as a means to offset the impact of the Social Security tax on low-income workers. A reduction in income-tax rates for the population at large in the Revenue Act of 1978 was similarly motivated, at least in part, to offset Social Security tax increases enacted the year before. And more recently, in the past two years, the reduction in the Social Security tax rate itself was intended to provide taxpayer relief to help with the recovery from the recent recession. Directly or indirectly, Social Security taxes have affected federal fiscal policy as a whole and, thus, how much revenue has been raised for the Treasury overall.

Whatever the lore that people want to cling to, Social Security is not the "golden boy" of federal finance. The program is part of what makes up the fiscal condition of the federal government and the declining circumstances it now finds itself in. In fact, this year, for the third year in a row, Social Security tax receipts are lower than the Social Security benefits paid out by the Treasury. And under current projections made by the Social Security Administration's actuaries and

CBO, the program's expenditures—absent corrective action by law-makers—will exceed its tax receipts for years to come.

Hence, a big-picture view of our fiscal condition is that nothing is sacred, not even Social Security.

What Matters Isn't the Trust Funds' Condition; It's How Social Security Affects the Government's Condition

What's confusing for the public is the difference between Social Security when considered in isolation and Social Security when considered as a part of the government. The language of the law requires an "actuarial evaluation" of the Social Security trust funds, and that's what drives the isolated view. From that perspective, the basic question is "Will there be a sufficient balance of securities posted to the trust funds—i.e., to convey sufficient *spending authority* to the secretary of the Treasury—to permit full payment of the future benefits that are scheduled?"

That evaluation is done annually by a board of trustees, comprised of three Cabinet officers, the commissioner of Social Security, and two public representatives, and it has historically been the main instrument for giving official Washington comfort or unease about Social Security's condition. At times it has prompted legislative expansions, at other times it's put on a damper, and on a few occasions it's even resulted in notable constraints.

Adding to that aura of independence is that non-partisan actuaries make the official estimates and are required to attest to the methods and assumptions for determining the program's "actuarial" condition. Taking direction on key variables from the trustees, they determine whether the program is in "actuarial balance" (a good condition), "actuarial imbalance" (a bad condition), or "close actuarial balance" (a not-too-bad condition). And the determinations are made for varying periods of measure, ranging from five years into the future at the earliest to 75 years at the longest. The degree of balance or imbalance is then calculated as an average for each of the periods evaluated, typically with a 5 percent tolerance as the trigger for a conclusion as to whether the system is in or out of balance. The calculation starts with the amounts recorded to the trust funds at the beginning of each period, followed by computations of income and disbursements, and ending with outcomes expressed as a percent of taxable payroll, as a percent of GDP, and even in present-value dollar-denominated terms to arrive at some measure of funded or unfunded liabilities. Adding to the endeavor, an evaluation is made using three different paths of future demography and economics: one rendering a more pessimistic outlook, a second rendering a more favorable one, and the third falling in between.

In the end, a complicated, multi-faceted test of actuarial soundness renders various measures of Social Security's projected financial condition, all of which leads to a single point of emphasis under the middle case of assumptions: *when will a trust fund of non-negotiable assets receiving non-negotiable interest from the Treasury be exhausted?*

For the layperson, that complexity overwhelms what should be straightforward. The process is arcane and impenetrable, and given the economic events threatening the nation's financial future, the conclusions rendered have repeatedly been of questionable value, certainly in recent years. For more than 20 years the trustees have been reporting large future problems. And by the nature of what has been evaluated—trust-fund balances—they have not portrayed any immediate threats. Thus, routinely dismissed as perils decades in the future, the adverse trustees' reports have done little to move lawmakers to take corrective action.[3]

---

3. Typically in the past, when lawmakers made assessments of Social Security's future condition, they focused heavily on whether the system's income and expenditures were projected to be in balance "on average" over the following 75 years. And usually it was the early decades in that period that made the "average" look good. The long-range outlook, influenced greatly by increasing longevity, a growing number of recipients, and rising real benefits, rarely looked favorable. But long-range projections are highly uncertain, and lawmakers routinely put particular emphasis on the 75-year "average"

FIGURE 3.1. Social Security Is Now Running Cash Deficits

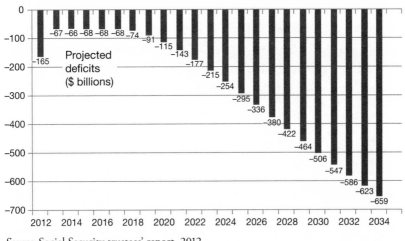

Source: Social Security trustees' report, 2012.

In contrast, from the perspective of Social Security as part of a larger government, what matters most is the financial condition of the government. A subsidiary of a major global company may take comfort that in the past it generated considerable profits for its owner, but if its parent company is now going deep into the red and that subsidiary is no longer generating profits, what does the past matter? How can the subsidiary that now generates losses survive if the parent company goes under?

Right now, there is more going out of the U.S. Treasury for Social Security than there is coming in. It's nice to know that there has been an accounting of what came in and went out in the past, but what matters most at this juncture is how much more is going out than

on the assumption that what really matters is what might happen in the nearer portion of the projection period, not three-quarters of a century away. Since the mid-1970s, the fact that the baby boomers born in the post–World War II period would deluge the program with their numbers and high cost early in the 21st century was routinely recognized but too far off to coax lawmakers to make changes in the program that would fully recognize the consequences of society's aging.

coming in and to what extent that will contribute to a rapidly escalating debt that threatens the nation's well-being.

Social Security taxes fell below Social Security expenditures beginning in 2010, when the shortfall was $51 billion. Last year, it was $148 billion; this year, $165 billion; and by 2025, nearly $300 billion. Thereafter, the shortfalls will grow increasingly larger, theoretically ending in 2033, when the Treasury will no longer be able to legally pay benefits in excess of tax receipts. The cumulative shortfalls from now through 2033 would total $5.7 trillion, and that assumes the Social Security tax cuts enacted for calendar years 2011 and 2012 are not continued in future years—a pretty dubious assumption given the difficulty lawmakers have in raising taxes once they put a cut in place.[4]

---

4. The Social Security tax cuts enacted for 2011 and 2012 reduced the tax rate from 6.2 percent to 4.2 percent on the employee side only (the employer side remains at 6.2 percent). Presumably, the lower rates would be in effect for those two years only. The two-year revenue loss for the Treasury is estimated to be $215 billion. The table in the text, based on projections in the 2012 Social Security trustees' report, assumes that the tax cut is allowed to expire at the end of 2012. Thus, the amount of the Social Security deficit shown in table falls from $165 billion in 2012 to $67 billion in 2013. If the tax cut is extended to 2013 and later years, the revenue loss will be much higher.

Four
THERE IS NO TIME LEFT TO PUNT AGAIN

The stress of entitlement spending has been on the policy blackboards of the past four Administrations and at least the last 10 Congresses. For the most part, with lots of rhetoric, feeble efforts, missteps, and no feeling of urgency, they have kicked the can down the road. Time, however, is no longer our friend. The fundamental choice in front of lawmakers now is whether to continue the political gridlock that

FIGURE 4.1. Taxes as Share of Economy, 1952–2011

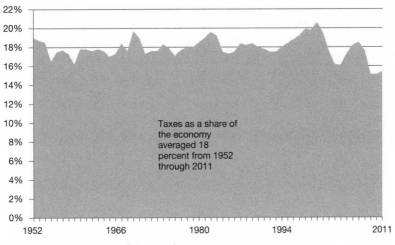

Taxes as a share of the economy averaged 18 percent from 1952 through 2011

Source: Economic Report of the President, 2012.

leaves us with the status quo and all its threatening consequences, or make the hard decisions that change the fiscal path we are on.

Confronting the mounting debt requires tackling the major cause of our rising expenditures: the uncontrolled spending we make for Medicare, Medicaid, and Social Security. Federal taxes cloud the picture. Yes, higher taxes could help contain the debt, but they could also impair economic growth. More to the point, beyond the immediate future, our troublesome outlook is not due to a potential loss of future tax revenue or an erosion of the tax base. It's about lots of new spending.

As a share of the economy, federal taxes have fallen over the past few years as a result of the recession, and they are relatively low today, taking a 15.7 percent bite out of the economy.[1] But even if they rose or were legislated back to where they've been for the past 60 years—averaging 18 percent—they would put only a modest dent in the escalating course of the national debt.[2]

---

1. During the 60-year period, federal taxes peaked as a share of the economy at 20.6 percent in 2000, and the lowest point of 15.1 percent occurred in 2009 and 2010. See "Economic Report of the President, 2012," Table B-79.

2. CBO's alternative long-range budget projections, which assume continuation of the Bush tax cuts and permanent relief from the alternative minimum tax for the next decade, show overall federal taxes rising to 18.5 percent of GDP by 2022 and leveling out thereafter. This is somewhat higher than the average of 18 percent over the 60-year period from 1952 to 2011. That higher level is not based on any detailed projections of federal tax provisions, but merely on the assumption that lawmakers would hold overall federal taxes at something close to the historical norm. Even with extension of the Bush tax cuts and continuing AMT relief, future taxes would continue to grow as a share of the economy because of "bracket creep." While the federal income-tax brackets for individuals are adjusted for inflation, historically wages have grown faster than inflation, and over time more of taxpayers' incomes fall into higher tax brackets. However, the 18.5 percent assumption is not a reflection of the effects of bracket creep, but a more generalized perspective reflecting the historical propensity of lawmakers to adjust federal taxation in one way or another to hold down the various automatic and ad hoc changes that would cause federal taxes to grow as a share of the economy.

FIGURE 4.2. The Rising Cost of
Maintaining a "Status Quo" Fiscal Path

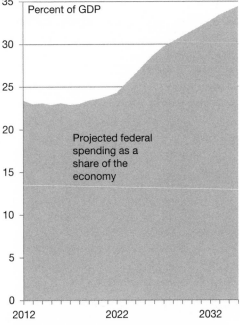

Source: Congressional Budget Office, 2012.

Over the next two decades taxes would have to rise 30 percent above their historical norm just to match the rising expenditures of the big three entitlement programs. If we procrastinate and wait two decades to raise them, CBO projects the interest cost on the accumulated debt would drive that figure up to 80 percent, and that assumes all other federal spending would fall.[3]

In effect, if we waited two decades to raise taxes, they would have to take a 33 percent bite out of the economy—i.e., one out of every three dollars of what's produced—to cover the total cost of government.

---

3. Calculations of potential future tax burdens used here were derived from CBO's alternative long-range budget projections.

To make a more poignant case, if the entire package of Bush-era tax cuts is allowed to expire (and no further relief provided from the "alternative minimum tax" for middle-income taxpayers), two decades from now taxes would still have to be set at a level equal to 30 percent of the economy to match the total cost of government.[4] That level of taxation—nearly double what it is today—would be unthinkable in terms of the burden it would place on the nation's workers.

And a bet that such tax increases would still reap benefits from a lower national debt would be an enormous gamble, in terms of the negative effect they could have on both economic growth and our ability to trade effectively in international markets. The world will likely be a much more competitive place then, as today's newly emerging economies grow into robust producers, and higher taxes will only add to the cost of the goods and services we produce.

FIGURE 4.3. Taxes Would Need to Double in 2032 to Match Projected Federal Spending (as a Share of the Economy)

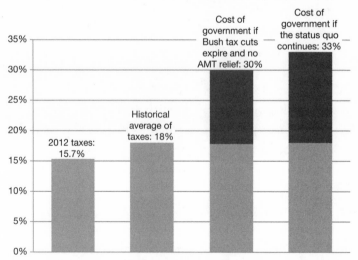

---

4. Under CBO's extended baseline projections—which assume expiration of the Bush tax cuts at the end of 2012 and no further relief from the alternative minimum tax—

The Hard Facts

A critical look at our deficits during the next decade is enlightening. Over the period from now until 2022, more than half of the post–World War II baby boomers will become seniors—defined here as reaching age 65. If we assume no changes are made to our fiscal path—just more of the status quo—persistent budget deficits could add nearly $14 trillion to our Treasury debt.[5] And spending for Medicare and Social Security for this period would exceed the taxes and premiums those programs generate by more than $6 trillion. Although those costs are primarily driven by Medicare, both programs would run deficits throughout the period and together would account for 40 percent of the projected rise in the debt.

The remaining portion is mainly the result of a $6 trillion run-up in the Treasury's interest costs on the debt, including a portion attributable to the Medicare and Social Security deficits. Together, those interest costs and the Medicare and Social Security deficits account for $12.2 trillion of an estimated $13.8 trillion in new debt that could accumulate by the end of 2022.

What this suggests is that the rest of the federal budget would have added only $1.6 trillion to the debt over that period. And this even assumes that Medicaid—as part of that all-other category—would

---

total federal tax revenues would equal 23 percent of GDP by 2032. (Note that in contrast, under CBO's alternative budget projections, taxes would equal 18.5 percent of GDP in 2032.) Absent changes in federal spending, overall primary expenditures would rise to 25 percent of GDP by then, and adding projected interest on the debt equal to approximately 5 percent of GDP would increase total federal spending to 30 percent of GDP.

5. The figures reflected here were derived from CBO's March 2012 alternative 10-year budget projections, which assume that the Bush tax cuts are continued and also that various other spending constraints required by law and routinely bypassed by Congress are overridden again throughout the coming decade. Although not assumed under CBO's projections, the figures in the text and table also assume that the Social Security tax cuts of 2011 and 2012 are continued throughout that period.

have grown from $258 billion in 2012 to $622 billion in 2022 and spent a total of $4.9 trillion. In effect, without the deficits of Medicare and Social Security, the spending on Medicaid, and the interest on the debt, the federal budget would be running a $3.3 trillion surplus over the 11 year period.

TABLE 4.1. Projected Federal Budget Deficits and Selected Contributors, Cumulative 2012–2022

	($ trillions)
Cumulative federal budget deficits for the 11-year period	13.8
Medicare and Social Security deficits, combined	6.2
Interest on federal debt	6.0
Subtotal	12.2
Remaining deficit	1.6
Remove Medicaid spending from remaining deficit	4.9
Surplus from all other government taxes and spending	3.3

Source: Calculations derived from CBO's March 2012 Budget Projections (alternative series), and the 2012 Social Security trustees' report (among other assumptions, the analysis here assumes continuation of 2011–12 payroll-tax cut).

In the decades to follow, pressure on the federal budget will rise as Medicare and Social Security expenditures continue to grow in excess of their tax and premium revenues. Measured in terms of today's economy, their combined annual deficits could climb to $1 trillion by 2035.

Society's aging is an issue that has long hovered over the federal budget. What's patently obvious from the numbers shown here is that the time has arrived when it can no longer be ignored.

TABLE 4.2. Projected Medicare and Social Security
Deficits, 2012–2035

Year	($ billion)*
2012	400
2020	700
2035	1,000

*Figures are rounded. The deficits shown for 2020 and 2035 were
adjusted to reflect what they would be if they occurred in 2012.
Source: Calculations derived from CBO's March Budget
Update and its 2012 Long-Term Budget Outlook, and the 2012
Social Security and Medicare trustees' reports. Among other
assumptions, assumes continuation of 2011–12 payroll-tax cut.

The secondary issue is the perplexing rise in the nation's health-
care costs, which will only amplify the federal spending driven by the
growing enrollment in the government's major health-care programs.

The Practical Window for Containing
the Nation's Health-Care Costs Starts with
Medicare and Medicaid

If we put aside political posturing by those who would protect government "entitlements" as a policy bias, it is the amalgamation of Medicare
and Medicaid into the nation's system of health-care delivery that gives
rise to the presumption that the only way to deal with the rapid rise
in their expenditures is through a broad national approach, not by
simply constraining their benefits. The thinking is that only through
a comprehensive system of financing and managing health care—a
national insurance program or some facsimile thereof—can health-
care costs really be reined in. The universe of health-care spending

is often analogized to a large balloon: if you squeeze it at one end, it will only expand at the other. As the reasoning goes, squeezing public funding (i.e., Medicare and Medicaid) will only put greater pressure on providers of service (hospitals and doctors), private insurers (thus raising the premiums the insured pay), and patients (forcing them to spend higher amounts out of pocket). In effect, the argument is that the amount spent on health care won't change.

Proponents of a universal approach contend that only an aggregated strategy linking health-care financing to how and what services are provided can compel measures that will eliminate waste and inefficiencies in the delivery of care (for instance, excessive testing and insurance paperwork), and force greater attention to outcomes that improve the effectiveness of medical treatment in the most economical manner. In short, they see it as the only way to really save money.

People have made that claim for years. But what comprehensive approach is there that the many factions can coalesce around? Can politically palatable policies actually be devised that affect the overall practice of medicine, or do we have to devise a single-payer system (a.k.a. national health insurance)? If so, how do we nationalize a massive complex of privately supplied, insurance-based health care: health-care companies, hospitals, skilled-nursing facilities, doctors, pharmaceutical makers, HMOs, medical-equipment manufacturers, and the many others with a stake in the health-care economy?

And if somehow we could, what would be the consequences? Can we avoid the queuing up and rationing that have plagued other countries with such a system? Can we avoid a decline in the quality of medicine and continue to encourage scientific and technological advancements that benefit us all? Can we continue to encourage the best and the brightest to choose medicine as a profession? And, obviously, will it go beyond theory and actually save money?

The nation's health-care system, with $2.8 trillion in expenditures, is larger than the gross domestic product of all but five other countries. It is a monolith of economic activity. How could we conceivably transition to some aggregated national system in a non-disruptive way? Add to this the politics of bringing together all those businesses and institutions with a stake in the system—the various trade and interest groups and the multitude of advocacy organizations, from AARP to the Chamber of Commerce—and the task becomes daunting. One can hypothesize that the only way to contain health-care costs is to attack the problem across the board, but fundamentally consolidating the means of financing and distributing our medical care may be little more than a fanciful aspiration by those yearning for nationalized medicine.

Medicare and Medicaid already provide large centralized devices for addressing the issue. True, they don't serve the entire population, and Medicaid policies do vary from state to state. But their recipient populations are huge, they permeate all facets of the health-care economy, and, most importantly, their policymaking is concentrated within the governmental bodies that fund them.

The federal government is the logical place to start for other reasons as well. All told, the feds finance directly or indirectly close to half of the nation's health-care costs (including other elements such as NIH research, veterans' and military care, and tax preferences for employer-provided health-insurance premiums and expenditures).

And while the rise in health-care costs is a broad phenomenon affecting all segments of the population, it is the aging of the population that is most problematic. It may be politically incorrect to say we should start with Medicare and Medicaid, but it is their recipient populations who consume the largest per capita share of the health-care dollar.

TABLE 4.3. Per-Enrollee Spending on Health Under
Medicare and Private Insurance, 2010

Medicare	Private health insurance
$10,600	$4,000

Source: Centers for Medicare & Medicaid Services, National Health
Expenditures, 2010 (Table 16).

The Need to Restore Price Sensitivity

The Centers for Medicare & Medicaid Services are already engaged
in studies and reforms that use national data to better identify and
reward the most effective treatments and best medical providers, to
change the fee-for-service payment structure to get the most bang for
the buck, and to use technology to manage personal health histories
and attack the maze of insurance rules and paperwork that plagues the
system. Not to diminish the ultimate utility of these reforms, but their
promise of rationalizing and containing the nation's spiraling health-
care costs is probably years away. And those approaches come at the
problem mostly from the provider side.

The inefficiencies of fee-for-service medicine being what they
are, perhaps one of the larger impediments to cost containment is
the absence of price sensitivity by both patients and providers. There
are few politicians who talk about the need to challenge the public's
insensitivity to the price of medical services. Bucking the "fix me at
whatever cost, my insurance will cover it" mind-set is a hard sell. The
doctor, wanting to do the most for his or her patients, wanting to
deflect the cost to some amorphous third party, or wanting to avoid
the risk of a malpractice claim, has little incentive to take the most
cost effective, least expensive approach. And while cure is the purpose,
payment is for the service, not the outcome.

There was a time when we treated spending on medical care dif-
ferently. But as third-party payments evolved and costs rose, out-of-
pocket spending dropped precipitously. In 1960, more than one out

FIGURE 4.4. The Amount of Health Care Paid Directly by Consumers Has Fallen Greatly Since 1960

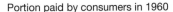

Portion paid by consumers in 1960   Portion paid by consumers in 2010

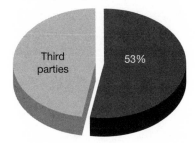
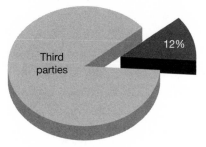

Source: Centers for Medicare & Medicaid Services, 2012.

of every two dollars spent on health care was paid directly by consumers—out of pocket. Today, that figure is a little more than one in 10.

Changing that mix in favor of more out-of-pocket spending is probably the most direct means of restoring price sensitivity to the patient-provider relationship. The closest some policymakers get to conceding this point is when they advocate limiting or eliminating the tax-exempt status of employer-provided health benefits. It would effectively force people to pay more for their health care because the benefits or health-insurance premiums their employers pay on their behalf would become taxable.[6]

Under Medicare and Medicaid, however, enrollees don't have tax preferences for whatever premiums they may pay. Thus, the only way to achieve greater price sensitivity is to limit the benefits directly. That obviously increases out-of-pocket spending, and as such it hits the decision-making process head-on about what the patient needs

---

6. Moving in that direction, the 2010 health-care legislation is scheduled to impose new taxes on so-called "Cadillac" health-insurance plans beginning in 2018, which may prompt some employers to reduce the scope of their plans. That may trim the fat from some overly generous plans and, where employees are given a choice of plans, motivate them to adopt insurance with greater out-of-pocket features—higher deductibles, co-payments, and the like.

and what the doctor provides. It would affect the behavior of both of them and, thus, the amount of health care consumed. It would affect the number of visits a patient seeks and a doctor prescribes. It would require deciding between the cheap test and the expensive one. It would require deciding between surgery and non-invasive treatments. It would require choosing between generic drugs and brand names. The balloon analogy ignores this.

That said, few politicians are yet willing to admit that sacrifice is necessary. For a politician, there is no upside in calling for large increases in cost sharing, deductibles, or co-insurance, for capping doctor visits or inpatient hospital days, for questioning the high cost of an expensive test over a cheaper one, or for limiting the number of tests or referrals. No politician is saying that more of your doctor's bill should be on your nickel, not your insurer's, not your employer's, not the government's. No one is pushing for greater out-of-pocket spending by consumers.

It's kind of a vicious circle. The payment of medical care by third parties is supposed to ease the burden of large health-care costs on consumers, but given the high price of even the simplest of medical services, how can you ask the consumer to pay more even if that ulti-mately would ease the price strains that inherently plague the system?

That condition being what it is does not diminish the need to take action. Abhorrent as such measures may be for lawmakers, the rising cost of health care demands attention. Restoring reality to the prices we pay for medical care is critical, but the trimming of Medicare and Medicaid benefits involves more than the question of whether and how it will alter the use of health-care services. Medicare and Medicaid spending is out of control, and the issue is as much about the need to save money, plain and simple. It's about where the money will come from to pay for their mushrooming expenditures and everything else we want the government to do.[7] And, most importantly, it's about

---

7. In the context of the 2009–10 health-care debate, see again "The Nation's Health Care Conundrum . . . ," Concord Coalition, loc. cit.

accepting the reality that our government's "debt bubble" cannot expand indefinitely.

Real Change Means Getting Back to the Purpose of Having Government-Financed Health Care

Whatever rationales people may have for containing Medicare and Medicaid spending, at a very basic level it means resurrecting the primary reason the government got involved in financing health care in the first place—i.e., to help ensure that the cost of medical care doesn't preclude access to it. And that calls for adopting new policies that aid those people most in need and that lessen the degree of financial support for those whose economic circumstances allow them to purchase other insurance or pay for their health care by other means, including out of their own pockets. To accomplish that requires measuring economic well-being—i.e., means testing—a process that now exists for those seeking assistance through Medicaid, but not Medicare, which is by far the larger spender on the aged population.

Outright means testing for Medicare eligibility—where people would have to divulge their income and assets to a government bureaucrat who would determine if a person qualifies and for how much—would be an obvious non-starter. No one would expect the government to set up a new apparatus of claims reviewers, probably numbering in the tens of thousands, to periodically examine the economic condition of nearly all of the nation's seniors. It is too intrusive, and there would be outrage. Even if adopted, it would be an administrative monstrosity.

In a number of less intrusive ways, Medicare already has various means-testing attributes. If the corollary of means testing is that well-off people pay more for coverage, that now occurs through the Medicare Hospital Insurance (HI) tax and the premiums Medicare enrollees pay for Parts B and D of the program (covering physician services and prescription drugs). The HI tax is levied on all earned income from work, but the package of HI benefits is the same for everyone when they become eligible. The fact that higher-income people pay more taxes during their working years does not mean they receive greater benefits when they retire. Means testing also emerges in the premiums that higher-income Medicare recipients pay for Parts B and D benefits. Enrollees with adjusted gross incomes above a certain level—in 2012, $85,000 for a single person and $170,000 for couples—must pay a higher premium than those with lower incomes, and like those who pay relatively large HI taxes, they don't receive greater Part B or Part D benefits. They simply pay more. It occurs at the lower end of the income spectrum too: under Part D, enrollees with limited assets and income are eligible for assistance to meet cost-sharing requirements for their prescription drugs. And it occurs as well with people who are eligible for both Medicare and Medicaid (who, by definition, have met a means test), or with those who are poor or near-poor, can't afford Medicare, and need help "buying into" Medicare or meeting the program's coinsurance and cost-sharing requirements. To varying degrees, state Medicaid programs subsidize those costs.

But what's absent from those provisions is cost containment. They suppose that well-off people pay more for their coverage and the less well off pay less, but they do little to restrain how much health care is consumed. Paying more taxes or premiums for Medicare as income rises does not directly diminish costs or use, since the higher amount people pay is not derived from how much health care they receive. Generally, most of what they pay occurs in their working years through the HI taxes they paid, long before they enroll in the program. And that in no way affects the aggregate amount of health care they can receive as retirees.

The issues of direct means testing notwithstanding, what would lower spending is a reduction in benefits based on people's income when they are retirees—the higher it is, the lesser their coverage. Excluding well-off people altogether is possible too, but that would truly vitiate the concept of insurance. Someone making a million dollars a year as a worker pays up to $29,000 annually in HI taxes ($36,000 starting in 2013).[8] Over a 40-year work history, that's a lot of money. Should they really get nothing when they retire? And what if the millionaire lost his or her fortune as he or she approached retirement or simply transferred it to heirs? Are they suddenly entitled? And then how do we treat someone who had modest income through most of his or her life but inherited a fortune at retirement? They paid less than the lifelong millionaire, but they did pay. Is it simply a matter of what they are worth when they hit age 65? What did all their years of paying Medicare taxes really mean?

Problematic? Yes. Means testing in the strictest sense is complicated.

The middle ground is to make all retirees responsible for more of their medical bills and to subsidize the poor. Whether by imposing higher deductibles and coinsurance, prioritizing what is and isn't covered, raising the Medicare eligibility age, or converting Medicare from a program that pays medical bills to one that supports the purchase of private insurance, control over spending needs to be established. It involves limiting the amount Medicare will pay and giving additional help through Medicaid or some other means to those who can't afford to cover the gaps. While controls on Medicaid spending are needed as well, low-income assistance is that program's function.

Certainly in today's polarized political climate, there should be no illusion about the prospects of retrenching on federal health-care entitlements. With current economic conditions being what they are and the real stress of accumulating too much debt not being immediately felt, it's hard to get the public behind it. The difficulty is with the middle of the pack. The rich may say it is unfair (they paid the most), but they may shrug and say they'll just buy what they need.

---

8. The higher amount will be the result of an increase in the HI tax rate for high-income workers enacted as part of the 2010 health-care legislation.

The poor may be unable to say the same, but for many of them, there's Medicaid. But for the mainstream middle, there's just pain. For them, there is a fine line between needing to seek care and needing to spend less.

That said, we face the same fine line with so much else we buy in life—we make economic trade-offs every day. Today's third-party health financiers—governmental and private insurers—make those trade-offs opaque for medical care. As a nation, we need to get back to what insurance is all about. We need health insurance to protect us from the real catastrophe, that life-changing event that strikes from an accident, illness, or chronic condition and has the potential to devastate personal wealth and well-being. We buy homeowners insurance primarily for the fire or other major calamity that destroys the home. With car insurance, we need to be able to replace the car if we total it. We need health-care consumers to have much more "skin in the game." We need to pay more at the front end. We need changes that take us back to the basics of insurance and perhaps restore price sensitivity in the medical care we seek.

Few would question that the poor and near-poor need a safety net. They need access to preventive and incidental care that they won't necessarily buy, and a catastrophic event for them exists at a much lower threshold than it does for middle- and higher-income people. But assuming that the only way to achieve that is to blanket massive federal spending across the entire income spectrum is wasteful.

Getting Real About Social Security Benefits

Two principal factors account for Social Security's rising expenditures: the aging of the population and a deliberate policy decision made in 1977 to automatically pay larger benefits to each succeeding generation of recipients as wages in the economy rise over time.[9] The goal of

9. Public Law 95-216, Social Security Amendments of 1977.

the 1977 changes was to ensure that the percentage of pre-retirement earnings replaced by Social Security would remain roughly the same through time.

Of those two factors, the more perplexing is the demographics— a growing number of recipients. In an analysis done in 2003, the Congressional Budget Office estimated that approximately 55 percent of the rise in Social Security's cost over the following 70 years would be due to an increase in the number of recipients and improvements in life expectancy. The remaining 45 percent came from a projected increase in the value of the benefits that results from tying them to future wage growth.[10]

While increasing life expectancy is a remarkable achievement of medical science, its significance for public institutions such as Social Security and Medicare—established in a much different era—has been largely ignored or deliberately set aside by policymakers. The

---

10. See "The Future Growth of Social Security: It's Not Just Society's Aging," CBO, July 2003. In a later analysis contained in CBO's 2011 "Long-Term Budget Outlook," the agency found that aging of the population was the dominant cause of the growth of both Social Security and the government's health-care entitlements from the current time through 2035. To cite the report:

> Two factors underlie the projected increase in federal spending on the government's major mandatory health care programs and Social Security: the aging of the U.S. population, which increases the number of beneficiaries in those programs, and rapid growth in health care spending per beneficiary. CBO calculated how much of the projected rise in federal spending for the health care programs and Social Security under the extended-baseline scenario is attributable to aging and how much is attributable to "excess cost growth"—the extent to which health care costs per enrollee (adjusted for changes in the age profile of the population) grow faster than GDP per capita. . . . Of the two factors, aging is the more important over the next 25 years. With the interaction allocated between the two, aging accounts for 64 percent of the total projected growth in spending on Social Security and the major mandatory health care programs by 2035, and excess cost growth accounts for 36 percent. . . . The greater importance of aging is not surprising given that the aging of the baby-boom generation will significantly expand the number of people participating in those programs.

rapid progress of medical science, industrial innovation, and techno-logical development, as well as the nature of the American workplace, greatly changed the face of society over the past 75 years, but public programs established to deal with conditions that prevailed in the early and middle parts of the last century have remained mostly immovable objects, unfazed by society's improving health and its changing demo-graphic composition.

Even if Social Security's costs were not a source of the coming stress on the federal Treasury, the increase in longevity since the program's inception and its built-in policy of ever rising benefits run counter to the basic precept on which it was founded: to provide a floor of protection for the aged. In 1940, less than 7 percent of the population was aged 65 or older, and a man retiring at that age then could expect to live 12.7 more years; a woman, 14.7 more years. Today, 13 percent of the population is 65 or older, and a man retiring at 65 can expect to live 18.8 more years and a woman 20.8 years. The Social Security trustees project that males born in 2075 will live 17 years longer than those born in 1940, and females 14 years longer.

However, the phenomenon that people are living longer and can potentially work longer has been largely overwhelmed by the improved economic well-being of the aged and the many incentives today to

TABLE 4.4. Life Expectancy

Year	Life Expectancy at Birth		Life Expectancy at Age 65 (Remaining Years of Life)	
	Males	Females	Males	Females
1940	70.4	76.3	12.7	14.7
2000	81.1	85.0	17.5	19.9
2025	83.4	86.9	19.8	21.7
2050	85.4	88.5	21.2	23.0
2075	87.1	89.8	22.5	24.1

Source: Social Security trustees' report, 2012.

retire earlier. More importantly for public policy, a retiree today can expect a retirement period that is 50 percent longer than that of someone who retired 75 years ago, a fact that has had little effect on the nation's lawmakers.

Left to function on autopilot as the sacred cow of public entitlements, Social Security has had little adjustment. The status quo has loomed large and has had a tenacious grip on the policymaking process. Under policies now in place, each succeeding group of future recipients can expect to receive benefits for increasingly longer periods of time—which translates into an increasingly greater amount of benefits over their lifetimes. When Social Security began paying benefits in 1940, people at age 65 could, on average, expect to get benefits for close to 14 years. In 2000, they could expect to get benefits for more than 18 years. And for those reaching age 65 in 2050, the figure could be 22 years. In other words, a man retiring in 2050 could expect to receive 23 percent more over his lifetime than someone who retired in 2000, and 70 percent more than someone who retired in 1940—simply because he will have a longer life span. For a woman, the increases would be 16 percent and 56 percent, respectively.

But because of benefit liberalizations over the years, even those numbers are low. Benefit levels have been raised very substantially in relative terms since the early years of the program, and in terms of their purchasing power, they are much higher today. And if it weren't for resource limitations, according to the Social Security trustees, the rise would continue indefinitely under the benefit rules now in place. An average wage earner retiring at age 65 in 2035 could expect annual benefits that have 23 percent more purchasing power than those of a similar worker retiring this year. For someone retiring in 2050, the purchasing power would be nearly 46 percent higher. The trustees' analysis further shows that the value of those future benefits as a replacement for past earnings would also be considerably larger— almost 30 percent larger—than when the baby boomers began entering the workforce in the 1960s. The average replacement rate for a median-wage earner retiring in the 1960s was 28 percent. Under the benefits scheduled in law for those retiring in 2025 and later, it will be 36 percent.[11]

TABLE 4.5. Rising Value of First-Year Social Security Benefits for Future Retirees

Median wage earner retiring at age 65 in:	Annual benefits in first year of retirement (adjusted for inflation)	Percent increase in purchasing power over that of worker retiring in 2012
1950	$4,368	—
1970	11,040	—
1990	15,328	—
2000	15,839	—
2012	17,534	—
2020	18,966	8%
2030	20,491	17%
2035	21,652	23%
2040	22,920	31%
2050	25,655	46%

Source: Social Security trustees' report, 2012.

When we couple those changes with increasing life expectancies, higher first-year benefits would compound into much greater benefits over the lifetimes of future retirees. CBO projects that people who retire in the 2020s could receive lifetime benefits that, on average, are 19 percent larger than they were for those who retired in the past 10 years. For those becoming eligible in the 2040s, benefits could be

---

11. For those baby boomers retired or retiring in the period prior to 2025, the replacement rates are even higher, ranging from 41 percent for those who retired at age 65 last year to 37 percent in 2024.

53 percent larger. And for those becoming eligible in the 2060s, they could be 114 percent larger.

TABLE 4.6. Rising Value of Lifetime Social Security Benefits for Future Retirees*

For those becoming eligible in the period from—						
2002–11	2012–21	2022–31	2032–41	2042–51	2052–61	2062–71
Lifetime benefits adjusted for inflation—in constant 2009 dollars						
154,000	174,000	183,000	197,000	236,000	278,000	329,000
Percent larger than benefits of retirees eligible in the 2002–11 period						
—	13%	19%	28%	53%	81%	114%

Note: *Benefits represent a median for all workers within each of the various age groupings.
Source: CBO, "Long-Term Projections for Social Security: An Update," August 2009.

Opening a productive dialogue with the public about Social Security requires unconventional wisdom. It requires admitting that the program's benefits are scheduled to grow automatically. If there were only one fact to get across—*by locking in place the full-benefit age for all future retirees, the program builds increases in lifetime benefits*—it might illuminate why Social Security is in trouble. If the public understood this one fact, and that this uncontrolled expansion of benefits is the cause of the program's future deficits, it would put the policy trade-offs in a much more meaningful light.

A Meaningful Solution for Social Security's Troubled Outlook Requires Being Candid About the Options

The basic options lawmakers have for resolving Social Security's financial problems mirror those for relieving the fiscal strains confronting the government as a whole—borrow more, increase revenue, or constrain spending—and their implications are no different.

A "solution" that simply amounts to running up the national debt would signal to increasingly wary financial markets that Washington has no intention of doing what is necessary to get its fiscal house in order. Choosing to raise taxes is certainly a stronger signal but is similar to borrowing in that it places a claim on the future earnings of today's children. And even assuming that future workers would be able to afford higher taxes, there is a more ethical reason to question such a move—it would be a decision by today's lawmakers to confiscate their children's economic progress. If future generations of workers want to absorb the higher costs of Social Security, it should be their decision, not the consequence of the current generation's refusal to plan responsibly for a problem it created and knows is coming.

In this regard it is worth noting that, while the aggregate federal tax burden has hovered around 18 percent of the economy since the 1950s, as a nation we are more than 2.5 times wealthier now than we were then.[12] This suggests a certain resistance among the American public to taxes much above that level for any extended period of time. Today's aging baby boomers certainly don't have a higher federal tax burden than their parents did three decades ago. It raises the question of how receptive future generations will be to a permanent level of taxation that is 40 to 50 percent higher than it has been for more than half a century.

Maybe they will be, but there is no guarantee. Thus, aside from the dubious generational ethics of deciding today how our children should spend their future earnings, a reliance on tax increases to fund enlarged Social Security benefits risks an intractable political dilemma for future lawmakers: choosing between potentially unacceptable levels of taxation or abrupt benefit cuts.

---

12. See "Economic Report of the President," 2012, Table B-31, the column showing per capita GDP in constant dollars. The comparison in the text is based on the change in per capita GDP from 1963 to 2011.

This leaves the third option: phasing in constraints on the growth of future benefits. There are numerous ways to accomplish this, many of which have been floating around Capitol Hill for years. Prominent among them would be to raise the ages at which full or reduced retirement benefits can be received—now 66 for full benefits (rising to 67 after 2022) and 62 for reduced benefits[13, 14]—or slowing the real growth in benefits by changing the way benefits are calculated. Studied and examined routinely by congressional committees and outside advisory groups, those proposals contain few mysteries. What has confounded and hampered their enactment is fear of a senior backlash and election-year reprisals.

Reform options that constrain the built-in growth of future benefits are often described as "benefit cuts," a politically caustic description

---

13. Two key ages are pertinent to the receipt of Social Security retirement benefits: the earliest age when benefits can be paid, which is 62, and the age at which "full" benefits can be paid, sometimes referred to as the "full-benefit age." For people born before 1938, the full-benefit age is 65. As a result of legislation enacted in 1983, for those born in 1938, that age will be higher as it phases up to 67 for persons born in 1960 and later. The higher age phases up in two steps: to 66, by two months a year for people born between 1938 and 1943, and to 67, by two months a year for those born between 1955 and 1960.

14. It should be observed that from 1940 to 1956 the first age of eligibility and the full-benefit age were the same: age 65. Legislation enacted in 1956 allowed women to get "reduced" benefits beginning at age 62; for men, "reduced" benefits at 62 commenced in 1961. The reduction for electing to get benefits before age 65—what is called an actuarial reduction—was intended to ensure that people receive approximately the same benefits over their lifetime as if they had waited until 65. As in the past, the reduction today is based on the number of months before the full-benefit age that a person elects to receive benefits. The term "full-benefit age" is somewhat of a misnomer, as by no means is it the usual age that people begin to receive benefits nor is it the largest amount they can receive. The vast majority of recipients elect to receive benefits at earlier ages. The term is similarly misleading in that higher benefits can be paid if people wait until later ages to collect benefits. The benefits paid at the full-benefit age represent those resulting from the basic calculation of benefits using a person's earnings history, i.e., before additional adjustments are made (up or down) for early or delayed retirement.

that fuels opposition by the nation's seniors largely by the inference that benefit checks for current recipients will be reduced. No major restraint option, however, would alter the benefits of current recipients.[15] Moreover, the Social Security benefits of future recipients can be reduced from projected levels without producing a "cut" relative to what today's recipients can buy with their benefits—i.e., a real cut. This is "economic speak" for saying that raising Social Security's retirement ages gradually or changing the way benefits are calculated will not necessarily reduce the value of future benefits below the levels that prevail for today's retirees.

Nor does it necessarily mean that the role of the program as a replacement for pre-retirement earnings will contract over time. With a hike in the various retirement ages, it's not the level of monthly benefits that's being changed but the number of years over which they will be received. Is having the program operate with better regard for the changes in life spans really a cut in benefits? If a man retiring at age 65 in 1940 could have been paid benefits for the same proportion of his life as is now projected for a 2050 retiree, his benefits would have started when he was 59, not 65. He would have had benefits for six additional years. It is disingenuous to suggest that the program's future role as a source of retirement income would shrink by asking future workers to receive benefits a few months or years later than their parents and grandparents, who had shorter lifetimes.

Finally, it is important to ask whether the supposed "constraint" is from the package of benefits arising from the current computation

---

15. One exception would be a proposal to revise the way inflation adjustments are calculated, including Social Security COLAs for both current and future recipients, which are now based on the Bureau of Labor Statistics' Consumer Price Index for Wage Earners and Salaried Workers (CPI-W). The CPI-W would be replaced by a so-called "chained" CPI, which makes a correction for overstating the rise of the cost of living because of consumers' changing what they purchase as the price of their accustomed goods and services rise. Although criticized by a few observers as a "benefit cut," it is more of a technical fix in the way inflation is measured.

rules or what the system can afford to pay. If benefits are not curtailed by the stress of financial markets objecting to our rising debt, it is widely acknowledged that, if the trustees' projections come to pass, the trust funds will go belly up (i.e., have run through their "spending authority") by the early 2030s and the incoming Social Security tax revenues will only be enough to pay 75 percent of what the benefit rules currently dictate. Thus, it is misleading to judge reform options against a benchmark that assumes the current system can deliver everything implied by its unfettered benefit rules. Curtailment of the large increases in lifetime benefits for future recipients that current rules would produce is hardly a cut if there isn't enough revenue to pay for them in the first place.

In this regard, if cutting benefits for current recipients is truly a line in the sand and lawmakers don't take action to curb the much larger ones for generations to come, current law already anticipates a sudden 25 percent drop in benefits in 2033 that would affect all recipients thereafter, including those who are now or will shortly come onto the rolls. Upwards of 55 million post–World War II baby boomers—those 68 and older then—would still be alive and on the rolls. Think of it: an 80-year-old born in the middle of the baby boom would have his or her benefits suddenly reduced by 25 percent in 2033.

Is that just drama? No, it's current law. The honest comparison of proposals to change Social Security should be to benefit levels that current law can deliver, not to those under rules developed 30 or more years ago and that call for ever rising benefits.

Media pundits say lawmakers would never let a sudden cut in benefits happen. But that's cop-out punditry. There is no genie in a bottle. What would be the alternatives in 2033? Raise payroll taxes suddenly by 33 percent? Borrow more? From whom?

If their point is that procrastination is not realistic, they're right. The current dilemmas in Greece, Spain, and Portugal paint a depressing picture of what that implies. But for the past two decades the Social Security trustees have warned 10 Congresses and four Administrations that troubles would emerge for the system some time in the 2030s. Lawmakers have taken no action. What do you call 20 years of avoidance? The "status quo"?

What exactly will future lawmakers do if the "status quo" persists?

Lawmakers Need to Judge the Merits of Allowing Large Uncontrolled Increases in Social Security Benefits Relative to Other Claims on the Economy

During Social Security's first 40 years, benefits were raised only as lawmakers saw the need and perceived that the resources would be there.[16] That's not the case today; benefit increases are automatic and the resources to fund them aren't there. Retaining or modifying future benefits means lawmakers need to exercise the discretion their voters gave them. They need to judge the merits of making sizable automatic transfers to the aged and disabled relative to other budgetary priorities and, ultimately, other claims on the economy.

In supplemental views, a number of members of a 1979 Social Security Advisory Council put it this way:

> At the levels of real income prevailing in the 1930s (or perhaps even the 1950s), it can well be argued that it was appropriate, indeed, highly desirable—perhaps even necessary for the preservation of our society—that government should, by law, have guaranteed to the aged and disabled and their dependents replacement income sufficient to avoid severe hardship, and to have required workers (and their employers) to finance this system with a kind of "forced saving" through payroll tax contributions. But as real incomes continue to rise, it is not easy to justify the requirement that workers

---

16. Notable in this regard is that the level of pre-retirement earnings replaced by benefits for average earners in the first three decades of the program were in the range of 15 to 30 percent. Those rates were considerably lower than ones that now prevail for today's retirees and would arise under current law for future recipients.

and their employers "save" through payroll contributions to finance ever higher replacement rates far above those needed to avoid severe hardship."

Those members stated further that

... future Congresses will be better equipped than today's Congress to determine the appropriate level and composition of benefits for future generations. . . . Congress might elect to give more money to certain groups of recipients than to others, or to provide protection against new risks that now are uncovered. But precisely because we cannot forecast what form those desirable adjustments might take, we feel the commitment to large increases in benefits and taxes implied under current law will deprive subsequent Congresses, who will be better informed about future needs and preferences, of needed flexibility to tailor Social Security to the needs and tastes of generations to come.[17]

Unfortunately, most people today don't understand how generous Social Security will be for future recipients. They assume those benefits will have the same value then as they do today—not more. Thus, the downside of proposing benefit constraints is that it is easy to demagogue. And whether politicians are spurred by demagoguery or not, the mere threat of exploitation explains their reluctance to suggest restraint.

Amending Social Security's future spending path may be politically hazardous and polarizing, but to maintain that there is a free lunch is a prescription for political entrenchment and eventual economic disruption. It solves nothing. The acknowledgment that difficult changes have to be made to fix the program is an essential first step in opening a real dialogue.

---

17. "Social Security Financing and Benefits, Report of the 1979 Advisory Council." See statement of Henry Aaron, Gardner Ackley, Mary Falvey, John Porter, and J. W. Van Gorkum, (U.S. Gov't. Printing Office, Washington, D.C., 1979).

Five

"THE MAN BEHIND THE TREE IS YOU AND ME"

FOR MANY YEARS much of the debate about the stress of our future entitlement promises has revolved around the question of how to establish claims on future resources, rather than on how to increase them. Scheduling future tax increases and relying on future government borrowing are different ways of extracting resources from the economy. They may have different effects about who pays, who receives, and how much more or less one pays or receives, but they do not answer the question of how to produce more. No matter how much nominal wealth can be traded or cashed in to provide healthcare benefits and retirement income to the aged, it is the total amount of goods and services that can be produced in the economy that will determine society's economic well-being and its capacity to deliver.

Lawmakers from both political persuasions contend that federal tax changes are probably needed—some want them raised, some want them lowered. What's "fair"—a largely subjective matter—often dominates the debate. But for purposes of containing the debt and putting us on a sustainable economic path, the important criteria are less about whether taxes are too high or too low or whether changes will raise or lower revenue, and more about how they will affect economic activity. Do they stimulate or impair investment in people, machines, technology, and education? Do they stimulate or impair risk taking? Do they stimulate or impair business creation? Do they encourage the accumulation of capital? A nation built on capitalism needs to have capital. Tax policy is not neutral on creating capital—it can stimulate or hinder its availability.

At the moment, large future consumption expenditures are built into our entitlement laws and pre-programmed to grow. To cover them as scheduled without borrowing, someone will have to pay. If not through greater payroll taxes, then it will likely be through higher income taxes or some other tax on what the nation produces. That inevitably triggers a debate about who is to bear these costs. As one version of the old saying goes, "We won't tax you, we won't tax me, we'll tax the man behind the tree."[1] Ultimately, however, we will all be the "man behind the tree." For it's not who may most bear the tax burden. If the projected expenditures materialize, there will be no escaping the burden imposed on the future economy, whatever its form.

These are confusing economic times. For much of the past half-century, we have been accustomed to hiding those burdens by borrowing more. But the potential magnitude of the government's debt is too big to ignore.

The dramatic actions taken over the past few years to shore up the world's financial systems and to soften the recession have shaken the conventional view of the economy's well-being and the government's fiscal condition. The idea that the federal Treasury, in the course of four years, could seek more than $5 trillion in new borrowing and swell an already large national debt would have seemed preposterous a decade ago. Moreover, given the conspicuous political gridlock in dealing with our budget dilemma, how much credence does the public now give to repeated prognostications by lawmakers that our future

---

1. A saying often attributed to former senator Russell B. Long of Louisiana, a long-serving chairman of the Senate Finance Committee.

deficits can be lowered with little disruption in our lives? If nothing more was accomplished by the failed machinations of lawmakers last year to address the issue, it brought the problem out of the closet. And the public's discomfort today is an obvious plus.

Our "aging" demographics and rising health-care costs are not just random assumptions in a budgeteer's tool chest. They have been building steadily. Yes, the projections are not derived from some clairvoyant insights about what the future will bring. It's possible, for instance, that market forces could someday bring health-care costs under control. But a realistic perspective recognizes that those costs have risen sharply for decades, and for the nation to plan for the future based on the hope of unprompted containment is a risky proposition.

What's needed today is a heavy dose of pragmatism. The federal debt now equals nearly 70 percent of what we produce each year, representing a rapid climb from 35 percent a decade ago. What will happen if it reaches 150 percent over the next two decades? It's like a family that doubles its mortgage without doubling its income. From an even broader perspective, our federal debt now equals 10 percent of the entire world's annual economic output. What will happen if and when it grows to 20 or 30 percent? And will the world even let us get there? How big is too big?

Today, 10 percent of your tax dollar goes to pay interest on the debt, or we borrow even more to pay it. If nothing is done to change course, within two decades 40 percent of your tax dollar could be needed to pay that interest. Or . . . what? Borrow more? Would you lend to a company with a ledger like that?

Budgeteers label entitlement spending as permanent and nondiscretionary outlays, but it is only as inevitable as we let it be. It was created by laws and can be amended by laws. We have a moment now, a narrow window of opportunity created by the conditions we find ourselves in. Our long-term economic outlook is predicated on issuing more debt—lots more debt. For policymakers to ignore that condition and the things that create it, or to pass the buck to future generations to make the hard choices, is simply irresponsible.

It's not courage to make clear what for decades was opaque. It's not courage to act responsibly and do what's seemingly hard. It's statesmanship. It's about the real job of legislating.

APPENDICES

Appendix 1
The National Debt

"The large amounts of federal debt that would accumulate under . . . CBO's long-term budget scenarios imply that the government would have to spend increasing amounts to pay interest on that debt. The growth of debt would lead to a vicious cycle in which the government had to issue ever-larger amounts of debt in order to pay ever-higher interest charges. Eventually, the government would need to adopt some off-setting measures — such as cutting spending or increasing taxes — to break the cycle and put the federal budget on a sustainable path.

"The government would have trouble issuing ever-increasing amounts of debt relative to GDP forever because there is a limit to the amount that savers want to save. If federal debt grew faster than the maximum rate at which savers were willing to acquire that debt (in the form of Treasury securities), government policies would be unsustainable."

Congressional Budget Office, January 2010

Note: In this document, the national debt, the public debt, and Treasury debt all refer to the portion of the federal debt held outside of government accounts (e.g., excluding the Social Security and Medicare trust funds and other internal accounts of the Treasury), what is often referred to as the "federal debt held by the public."

TABLE 1A.1. Holders of the National Debt, 2004 and 2012*

	End of 2004		In 2012	
	Debt ($ billions)	Percent of total debt	Debt ($ billions)	Percent of total debt
Total national debt	4,408	100	10,554	100
Amount in U.S. hands	2,559	58	5,454	52
Amount in foreign hands:				
China	223	5	1,179	11
Japan	690	16	1,096	10
Oil exporters	62	1	265	3
Brazil	15	a	226	2
Caribbean Banking centers	51	1	224	2
Taiwan	68	2	178	2
Switzerland	42	1	148	1
Russia	**	**	142	1
All other	686	16	1,642	16
Total foreign	1,849	42	5,100	48

Notes: *As of February 29, 2012.
**Under $10 billion; counted in "all other."
aLess than 0.5%.
Source: Department of Treasury, April 2012.

Even after the nation fully recovers from the recent recession, federal budget deficits would persist under current policies, and the national debt would rise indefinitely.

FIGURE 1A.1. The National Debt, 2011–25

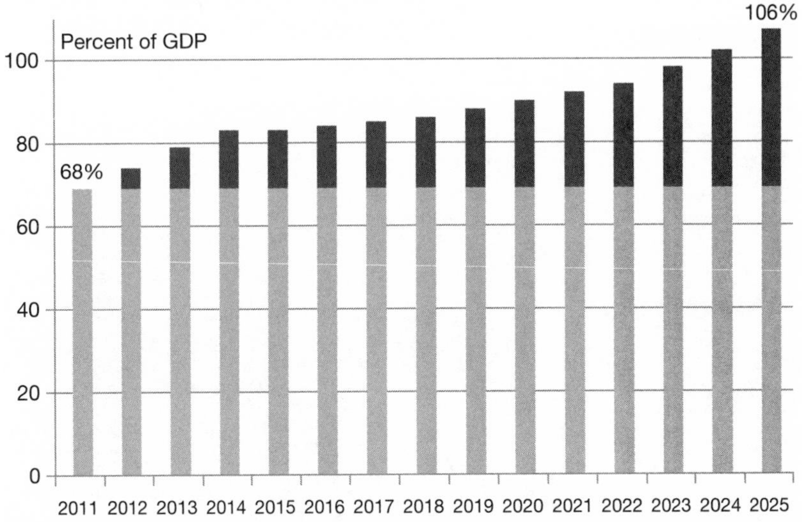

Source: Congressional Budget Office, 2012.

Gross domestic product (GDP) is an economist's term used to delineate the size of the economy. GDP represents the total output of goods and services produced, typically in annual terms. This year it is estimated to be $15.7 trillion. Under what are labeled baseline budget projections, the Congressional Budget Office (CBO) estimates that the national debt would fall from a level equal to 73 percent of GDP this year to 64 percent in 2020, and decline modestly thereafter. Under what CBO considers a "status quo policy" path, the debt would rise to 89 percent in 2020, 106 percent by 2025, and 200 percent by 2038.

Without remedial action by the President and Congress, the national debt could very well grow to an unsustainable level.

FIGURE 1A.2. The National Debt, 1972–2037

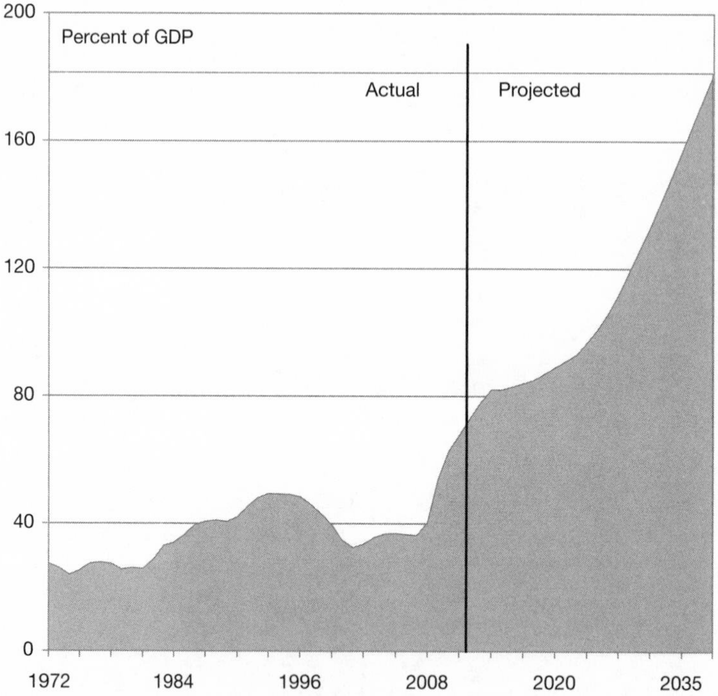

Source: Congressional Budget Office, 2012.

By the end of 2012, the national debt could reach a level equal to 73 percent of what the nation produces this year. That's almost three times what it was in 1980, and higher than at any point in the past 60 years. If that appears large, over the next 25 years, CBO projects, the debt, absent remedial measures, could rise nearly three-fold to a level of nearly 200 percent of what the nation would produce then. And interest on the debt then would be the equivalent of almost half of what the entire budget is today.

Appendix 2
The Federal Budget

FIGURE 2A.1. Projected Federal Revenues, Spending, and Deficit, 2012

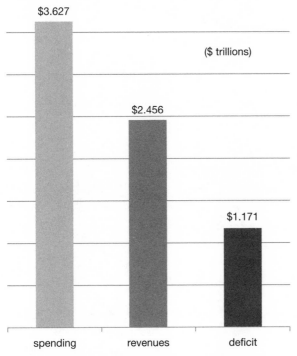

Source: Congressional Budget Office, March 2012.

FIGURE 2A.2. Medicare, Medicaid, and Social Security Spending as a Share of the Federal Budget, 2012

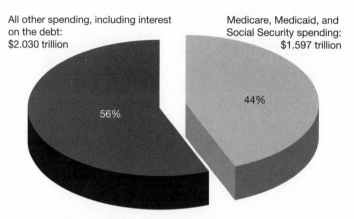

All other spending, including interest on the debt: $2.030 trillion

Medicare, Medicaid, and Social Security spending: $1.597 trillion

Source: Congressional Budget Office, March 2012.

FIGURE 2A.3. How the Share of Federal Spending for Medicare, Medicaid, and Social Security Has Changed

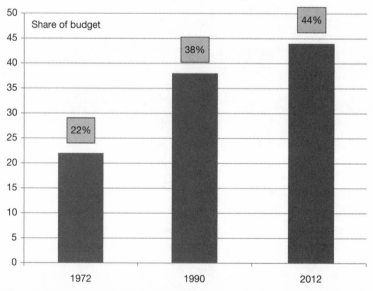

Source: Congressional Budget Office, March 2012.

Appendix 3
The Potential Consequences of Our Current Fiscal Path

- Much greater reliance on foreign nations to lend money to our Treasury (foreign investors now hold almost half of our national debt; one-fifth is held by China and Japan alone).

- If a point is reached where investors are unwilling to lend us money, an unprecedented financial crisis will occur—perhaps a meltdown.

- Soaring interest rates.

- A much larger tax burden on future generations.

- Economic stagnation or decline.

- Falling personal incomes.

- An eroding standard of living.

Appendix 4
Perceptions, Misperceptions, and Myths About the Problem

Common Perceptions	Reality Check
The problem is the result of . . .	
too much waste, fraud, and abuse, government mismanagement, and illegal immigrants' misusing social programs.	There have been many reports of wasteful government spending, mismanagement, and the misuse of social programs, and reducing these things can help address the long-term fiscal problem, but the larger causes are the effects of society's aging and the rising cost of medical care on major federal entitlement programs.
Too much revenue is lost from . . .	
the Bush-era tax cuts, corporate tax loopholes, and the "well-to-do" not paying enough taxes.	Adverse long-term fiscal problems were projected long before the Bush era. But even if the Bush tax cuts expire next year, the long-term problem would still be extremely large. Closing corporate tax loopholes and increasing taxes on the rich could be part of a remedy, but neither by itself created the problem and neither would fix it.

(continued)

Common Perceptions	Reality Check
The problem is caused by . . .	
the cost of two wars and the government's corporate bailouts.	The wars in Iraq and Afghanistan and the government's recession-driven efforts to assist corporations and large financial institutions are very expensive and contributed to the national debt, but they are largely onetime or temporary expenditures and pale in comparison to the effects of the future protracted rise of federal entitlement spending.
The problem is a myth:	
It is a conservative ruse to dismantle government programs, the underlying assumptions about the future are too pessimistic, the problem is the result of the recent recession, we can eventually grow our way out of it, and we've run deficits for decades—there's never been a meltdown.	Long-range budget problems have been projected for many years by both Democratic and Republican administrations, as well as by prominent economists and non-partisan analysts and institutions. The projections and concerns they evoke have long preceded the recent recession. The assumptions that underpin future projections have been examined and re-examined by professional actuaries and other experts, and while differences have emerged, they have been at the margins. The consensus by both liberal and conservative observers is that an unsustainable problem is coming and that it's not too far off.

Appendix 5
Why the "Problem" Is a Problem

The population is aging.

Over the hundred-year period from 1950 to 2050, the aged population (persons aged 65 and older) is projected to grow from 13 million to 84 million, and their share of the population will rise from one in 12 in 1950 to one in 5 in 2050.

FIGURE 5A.1. The Aged Share of the Population, 1950–2050

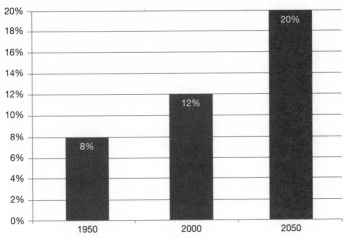

Source: Social Security trustees' report, 2012.

And dramatic strides have been made in lengthening life spans.

Over the 20th century, improvements in medical science (e.g., treating heart disease), changing lifestyles (e.g., reduction in smoking), and better working environments (e.g., less exposure to toxic and harmful conditions) have greatly extended the latter portion of peoples' lives.

In 1940, a man who reached age 65 could expect to live almost 13 more years; a woman, almost 15 more years. In 2050, the years of life remaining for a man at 65 is projected to rise to 21; for a woman, the number is 23. On average, people who reach age 65 now are living more than five years longer than those of the same age in 1940. By 2050, that number could rise to more than eight years. In effect, a person's potential retirement years are close to 40 percent longer today than they were in 1940, and could be 60 percent longer by 2050.

FIGURE 5A.2. Remaining Years of Life on Reaching Age 65

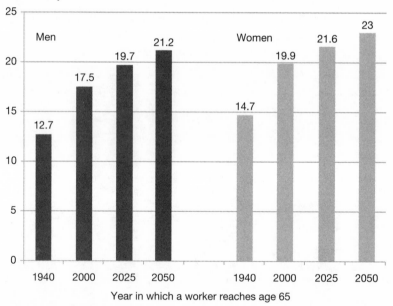

Source: Social Security trustees' report, 2012.

The baby boomers are reaching their senior years, and over the next 13 years, the number of people aged 65 or older will rise by 50 percent.

TABLE 5A.1. Growth of the Aged Population Compared to that of the Total Population, 1950–2035

Growth of the Population Aged 65 and Older		Growth of the Nation's Total Population	
(millions of people)		(millions of people)	
1950	13	1950	160
1975	23	1975	224
2000	36	2000	288
2012	43	2012	320
2025	65	2025	357
2035	78	2035	381

Note: Tables derived from Social Security trustees' report, 2012.

During the same period, the total population will grow by only 12 percent. Thus, where the aged represent 13 percent of the total population today, they will represent 18 percent in 2025 and 20 percent by 2035.

And the nation's birth rate has leveled off.

TABLE 5A.2. The Nation's Birth Rate Rose and Later
Declined in the Post–WW II Period

Year	(average number of births per woman in her lifetime)	Year	(average number of births per woman in her lifetime)
1940	2.23	2000	2.05
1950	3.03	2012	2.04
1960	3.61	2025	2.03
1975	1.77	2050	2.00

Source: Social Security trustees' report, 2012.

The baby boom was a temporary phenomenon for about 20 years in the middle of the last century. While birth rates tend to rise and fall over time, projections assume that future birth rates will cluster around the level of zero population growth, or two births per woman in her lifetime.

Thus, with the surge in the number of aged and a more modest birth rate, the future workforce is projected to grow more slowly, and the economy will likely expand at a slower pace.

The real growth of GDP equals the combined growth rates for total employment, productivity, and average hours worked. For the 58-year period from 1950 to 2008, the average growth rate in real GDP was 3.3 percent. In future years, the economy's annual growth rate is projected to be one-third to one-half lower. Much of the projected decline is attributable to slower growth in total employment.

TABLE 5A.3. Real Growth in GDP*
(Annual Rise in Percent)

1950–2008	3.3
1950–1960	3.5
1960–1970	4.2
1970–1980	3.2
1980–2000	3.3
2020	2.6
2030	2.1
2040	2.3

Notes: Figures are adjusted for inflation.
*Historical figures are from "Annualized Growth Rate and Graphs of Various Historical Economic Series," by Lawrence H. Officer and Samuel H. Williamson, *Measuring Worth,* 2009.
Source: Congressional Budget Office, 2012.

Consequently, the number of workers for every aged person could fall sharply. In 2035, the number of workers for every aged person could be nearly half of what it was in 1975.

FIGURE 5A.3. Number of Workers for Every Aged Person in the Population

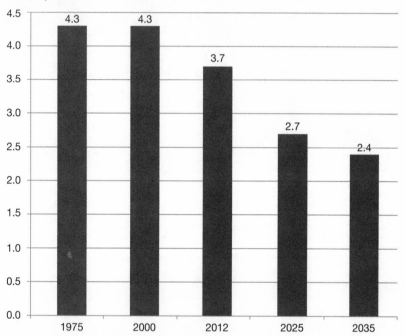

Source: Social Security trustees' report, 2012.

And the number of workers financing the benefits of each person enrolled in federal entitlement programs is likely to fall.

TABLE 5A.4. Number of Workers per Social Security Recipient, 1950–2050

Year	Workers Covered by Social Security	Number of Workers per Social Security Recipient
	(millions)	
1950	48	16.5
1975	100	3.2
2000	155	3.4
2025	178	2.3
2050	200	2.0

Source: Social Security trustees' report, 2012.

The number of workers paying into Social Security more than tripled from 1950 to 2000. It is expected to grow by only 33 percent from 2000 to 2050.

Where there were more than three workers for every Social Security recipient in 1975, there could be as few as two in 2050. Though the economy is projected to be larger 50 years from now, the redistribution of resources from workers to retirees could ignite generational strains.

Health-care spending has grown faster than the economy for decades.

> For the period from 1975 to 2007, per-person health-care spending (public and private) grew nearly 50 percent faster than the economy. While representing about one out of every six dollars of the goods and services the nation produces today, health-care consumption could account for more than one-fourth of the economy by 2035.

Even assuming that the rise in health-care spending moderates, CBO projected three years ago that the aggregate bill for the nation's medical care could someday account for as much as 40 percent of the economy, much of the increase driven by the rising health-care needs of the elderly.

While increases in longevity may lead to longer work lives, the incidence of diseases that affect the aged—who, on average, are the largest consumers of health care—are likely to rise as well. Among them are heart disease, Alzheimer's and other forms of dementia, diabetes, osteoporosis, and arthritis.

By some estimates, the number of people diagnosed with arthritis is projected to increase from 48 million in 2005 to nearly 67 million by 2030 (affecting perhaps 25 percent of the adult population).[†]

The number diagnosed with diabetes is projected to increase 165 percent, from 11 million in 2000 to 29 million in 2050. The largest rise will be among those aged 75 years and older (where the prevalence rises by 271 percent in women and 437 percent in men).[††]

FIGURE 5A.4. Causes of Death Among the Aged, 2006*

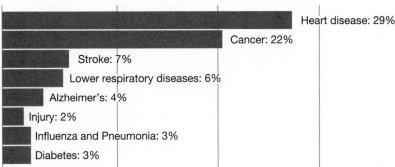

Heart disease: 29%
Cancer: 22%
Stroke: 7%
Lower respiratory diseases: 6%
Alzheimer's: 4%
Injury: 2%
Influenza and Pneumonia: 3%
Diabetes: 3%

[†]"Projections of U.S. Prevalence of Arthritis and Associated Activity Limitations," by Jennifer M. Hootman and Charles G. Helmick, Centers for Disease Control and Prevention, Atlanta, Georgia, 2005.

[††]"Projection of Diabetes Burden Through 2050 (Impact of Changing Demography and Disease Prevalence in the U.S.)," by James P. Boyle, Amanda A. Honeycutt, K. M. Venkat Narayan, Thomas J. Hoerger, Linda S. Geiss, Hong Chen, and Theodore J. Thompson, 2010.

*The CDC chart regarding causes of death among the aged does not add as the smaller "all-other" causes are not shown. As a group, the "all-other" category comes to 26 percent of total.

Source: Centers for Disease Control, 2006.

By some measures, the health-care expenses of elderly people are three to five times higher than those for younger people.

TABLE 5A.5. Personal Health-Care
Spending by Age, 2004*

Spending per capita by age group		
65+	Working age	Children
$14,797	$4,511	$2,650

*"U.S. Health Spending by Age, Selected Years
Through 2004," *Health Affairs,* November 2007.

FIGURE 5A.5. Share of Every $100 in the Economy Going Toward Health Care

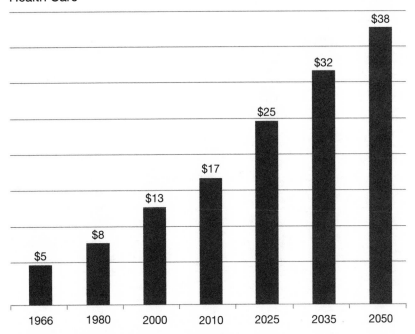

Source: Congressional Budget Office, 2009 and 2011.

As national health expenditures have risen, so has the federal government's share. Federal expenditures from the Treasury and health-care tax exclusions and deductions for employers and individuals together account for close to half of how the nation pays for its medical care today.

By far the largest sources are through Medicare and Medicaid (a portion of which is financed by the states). The share of the nation's total health-care bills paid by the two programs rose from 27 percent in 1980 to an estimated 39 percent in 2012.

TABLE 5A.6. Medicare and Medicaid's Rising Share
of Health-Care Spending

Year	National Health-Care Spending as a Share of GDP	Medicare and Medicaid's Share of the Nation's Total Health-Care Spending
1966	5%	8%
1980	9%	27%
2000	14%	33%
2012	18%	39%

Source: Centers for Medicare and Medicaid Services, National Health Expenditures, 2012.

FIGURE 5A.6. Federal Health-Care Entitlements' Growing Share of the Economy

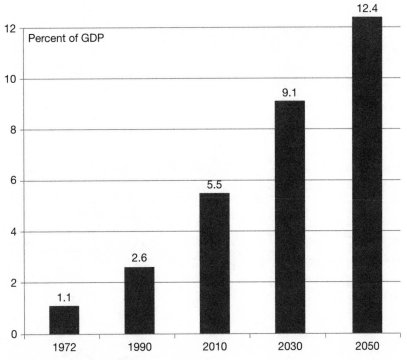

Source: Congressional Budget Office, 2012.

Spending for programs serving the aged, particularly Medicare, Medicaid, and Social Security, will rise rapidly.

Today, Social Security is the largest of the major federal entitlement programs. By 2034, Medicare will be the largest.

FIGURE 5A.7. Spending for Medicare, Medicaid, and Social Security, 2012–2050

	2012	2020	2030	2050
	(percent of GDP)			
Medicare	3.7	4.2	5.7	8.1
Medicaid*	1.7	2.8	3.4	4.3
Social Security	5.0	5.3	6.0	6.1
Total	10.4	12.3	15.1	18.5

*Also includes SCHIP and new exchange-subsidy spending.
Source: Congressional Budget Office, 2012.

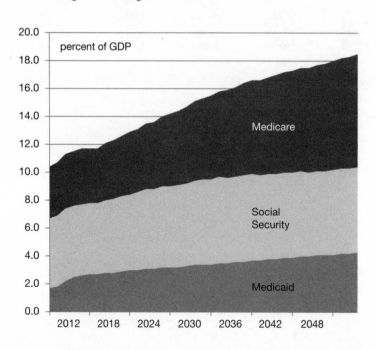

The aging of the population, notably as the baby boomers move into their senior years, is the most immediate driver of the growth of Medicare, Medicaid, and Social Security. Their looming enrollment will greatly expand the number of people being served.

FIGURE 5A.8. Effect of Aging and Rising Health-Care Prices on Spending for Medicare, Medicaid, and Social Security, 2012–2035

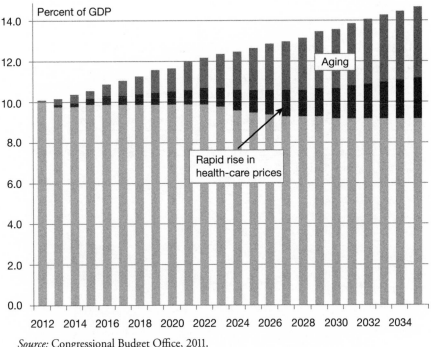

Source: Congressional Budget Office, 2011.

Aging versus rising health-care prices?

Either factor alone would boost spending, but the two together have a compound effect, causing spending to rise even faster. Aging is the more important factor over the next 25 years, as the baby boomers significantly increase the number of program recipients. It accounts for about 64 percent of the projected growth of the three programs by 2035.

TABLE 5A.7. Causes of Spending Growth of Medicare, Medicaid, and Social Security

	Percent attributable to:	
	aging of the population	rising health-care costs
By 2035	64	36

Source: Congressional Budget Office, 2009.

By far, the largest growth in spending by these three programs will be for health care.

TABLE 5A.8. Relative Growth in Spending Attributable to Medicare, Medicaid, and Social Security, 2009–2035

(source of growth in percent)	
Medicare and Medicaid	80
Social Security	20

Source: Congressional Budget Office, 2009.

Between now and 2035, four-fifths of the growth in spending by these three programs will be in Medicare and Medicaid.

Because of this growth, federal spending will increase faster than tax revenues, the interest expense of borrowing money will rise sharply, and budget deficits will persist and grow larger over time.

TABLE 5A.9. Federal Budget Revenues, Spending, and Deficits, 2012–2042

	(in percent of GDP)			
	2012	2020	2035	2042
Spending	23.4	23.6	34.4	38.6
Revenues	15.7	18.3	18.5	18.5
Deficits	−7.7	−5.3	−16.0	−20.2
Federal debt as a percent of GDP	63	89	181	247

Source: Congressional Budget Office, 2012.

Historically, federal taxes have equaled about 18 percent of GDP. CBO's projections assume taxes will rise modestly to 18.5 percent of GDP by 2022 and remain at that level thereafter. In 2012, the federal deficit is projected to equal 7.7 percent of GDP. By 2042, total federal spending could reach a level equal to 38.6 percent of GDP, and the deficit would equal 20.2 percent.

Medicare, Medicaid, and Social Security spending equals 10.4 percent of GDP today, and accounts for just under half of all federal budget expenditures other than interest on the debt. By 2042, it could reach a level equal to 17.3 percent of GDP. By 2050, it could reach 18.5 percent of GDP, an amount that by itself would equal the government's entire tax base.

FIGURE 5A.9. Federal Deficits, 2012–2042
(Amount of Spending in Excess of Tax Revenues)

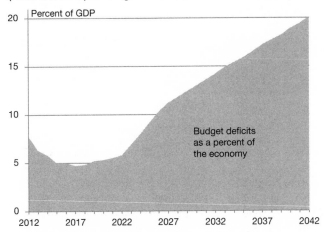

Source: Congressional Budget Office, 2012.

Federal expenditures (excluding interest on the debt) are referred to as "primary spending." Medicare, Medicaid, and Social Security's share of primary spending is projected to rise from 47 percent today to 67 percent in 2050.

TABLE 5A.10. Shares of Primary Spending Under the Federal Budget (Excludes Interest Costs)

	(percent)		
	2012	2035	2050
Medicare, Medicaid, and Social Security	47	62	67
All other spending	53	38	33

Source: Congressional Budget Office, 2012.

Projections of primary federal spending show the federal budget would run long-range deficits even if rising interest costs were not a factor.

TABLE 5A.11. Primary Spending and Revenues Under the Federal Budget (Percent of GDP)

	2012	2035	2042
Primary spending	22.0	25.8	26.8
Revenues	15.7	18.5	18.5
Primary deficits	6.3	7.4	8.3
Interest expenditures (excluded above)	1.4	8.6	11.8

Source: Congressional Budget Office, 2012.

FIGURE 5A.10. Federal Deficits Resulting from
Primary Spending, 2012–2050 (Amount of Primary
Spending in Excess of Tax Revenues)

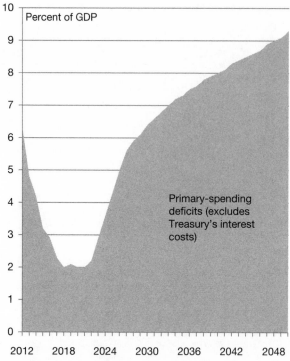

Source: Congressional Budget Office, 2012.

Reductions in "all-other" federal spending (i.e., other than Medicare, Medicaid, Social Security, and interest on the debt) can help remedy the problem, but this all-other category is not projected to be a major factor in driving up long-range federal spending.

TABLE 5A.12. "All-Other" Federal Spending (i.e., Other than Medicare, Medicaid, Social Security, and Interest on the Debt)

	2012	2025	2050
	(percent of GDP)		
Discretionary spending and other entitlements	11.6	9.1	9.3

Source: Congressional Budget Office, 2012.

In 2012, a little more than half of all federal spending went toward programs other than Medicare, Medicaid, and Social Security and interest payments on the debt. This category of all-other spending includes discretionary programs, which are funded through the annual appropriation process, and smaller entitlement programs (other than Medicare, Medicaid, and Social Security), which are usually funded according to the underlying statutes that establish eligibility and payment standards. Like Medicare, Medicaid, and Social Security, these other entitlement programs (e.g., unemployment insurance, SSI, etc.) are often referred to as "mandatory spending," since Congress generally has made funding available to them on a continuing or indefinite basis.

FIGURE 5A.11. Discretionary Spending and Other Entitlements, 1972–2050

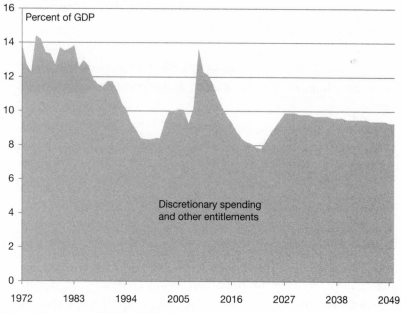

Source: Congressional Budget Office, 2012.

Interest payments on the national debt are a "virus" in the long-range fiscal outlook.

Under CBO's projections, the interest obligations accrued on the rapidly rising debt would eventually grow from 1.2 percent of GDP this year to 4.6 percent in 15 years and to 13.5 percent in 2050. The significance of this growth is illustrated by the fact that if Treasury's interest obligations were to reach 4.6 percent in 2025, they would be the equivalent to nearly half of today's combined spending for Medicare, Medicaid, and Social Security. The 2050 figure would be more the half of today's entire federal budget.

TABLE 5A.13. Comparison of Deficits Resulting from Primary Spending to Total Deficits, Including Interest Expenditures

	2012	2035	2042
	(percent of GDP)		
Deficits from primary spending	6.3	7.4	8.3
Add interest	1.4	8.6	11.8
Total deficits	7.7	16.0	20.2

Source: Congressional Budget Office, 2012.

FIGURE 5A.12. Comparison of Primary-Spending Deficits to Total Deficits, Including Interest Expenditures, 2012–2050

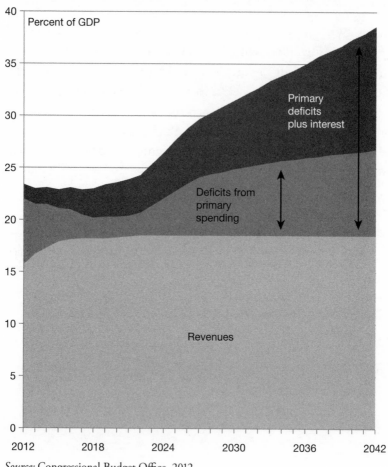

Source: Congressional Budget Office, 2012.

Appendix 6
The Significance of Addressing the Problem Sooner Rather than Later

Although the recovery from the recent recession may require that efforts to address the future fiscal gap be deferred, the earlier those actions can be implemented, the smaller the spending reductions and revenue increases we would need to achieve some measure of long-range fiscal stability.

The longer that policy action is put off, the more costly and difficult it will be to resolve. Delays in taking action would create three major problems:

• The amount of government debt would rise, which would displace private capital (reducing the total resources available to the economy) and increase borrowing from abroad.

• The share of federal outlays devoted to paying interest on the federal debt would grow, and policymakers would be less able to pay for other national spending priorities and would have

(continued)

less flexibility to deal with unexpected developments (such as a war or recession). Moreover, rising interest costs would make the economy more vulnerable to a meltdown in financial markets.

• The longer that action was put off, the greater the chance that policy changes would ultimately occur suddenly, possibly creating difficulties for some individuals and families, especially those in or near retirement.

Congressional Budget Office, 2009

Appendix 7
What Options Are There to Address the Problem?

The following is a list of some of the major options to address the long-range fiscal problem.

Medicare and Medicaid Options

1. Convert Medicare to a "premium support" program

Medicare is a program in which the federal government pays much of the cost of medical services used by enrolled recipients. Under this option, the federal government would provide enrollees with a fixed amount of money that they could then use to purchase health insurance in the private market. To reduce spending the level of the payment could be set at a percentage below the total expected medical costs per enrollee.

2. Limit growth of payment rates to Medicare providers

Medicare outlays are a product of the reimbursement rates for health services and the amounts that they are utilized. As such, spending could be reduced through across-the-board cuts in reimbursement rates. The cuts, to be determined by lawmakers, would decrease projected spending levels, affecting hospitals, doctors, and all other providers of health care.

3. Convert Medicare to a means-tested program

Currently, Medicare is not means-tested—i.e., eligibility is not limited by income or assets—and thus is available to all citizens and legal permanent residents aged 65 or older, provided they have worked for at least 10 years. Disabled individuals and those with permanent kidney failure are also eligible. This option would phase in a restriction on Medicare eligibility to only low-income or disabled individuals.

4. Increase Medicare out-of-pocket cost sharing

Under the current fee-for-service Medicare structure, there are different copayments and deductibles for different services. This option would create a single yearly deductible and copayment framework for all services under Medicare parts A, B, and D (see the following section on Supplementary Material for an explanation of these components). To reduce expenditures, the average enrollee's out-of-pocket payments would increase from the current level of approximately 10 percent of the cost of covered services to some higher level to be determined by lawmakers.

5. Raise the age at which Medicare eligibility begins

Currently, individuals are eligible for Medicare coverage at age 65, unless they receive coverage earlier because of a disability or one of a list of specific covered conditions, such as end-stage renal disease. This option would gradually increase the eligibility age to 67—which under current law is the eventual "full benefit" age for Social Security—and would continue to increase it in subsequent years as life expectancy rises.

6. Limit federal funding in Medicaid

Medicaid is a state-run program that is jointly funded by the federal government and the states. States determine who is eligible for Medicaid, and eligibility requirements vary across states and different groups of people (such as pregnant women or single men). The federal government pays a percentage of a state's total Medicaid costs, based on the state's per capita income. This option would establish a threshold at 100 percent of the poverty level, beyond which there would be no federal matching. In other words, any state spending on individuals at or below this threshold would be matched by federal spending (at a rate determined by per capita income in that state), and any state spending on individuals above that threshold would be entirely state-financed.

7. Medicaid block grants to states

Medicaid services fall into two categories: acute care (for hospital stays and physician visits) and long-term care (for nursing-home care and community-based assistance). The federal government pays a percentage of a state's total Medicaid costs, based on the state's per capita income. This option would convert the federal government's funding from a percentage to a fixed annual allotment for acute services and a continued percentage subsidy of long-term-care spending. The allotment would equal the level of Medicaid spending on acute care in 2012 indexed to inflation. In exchange for less funding, states would have more discretion regarding the operation of the program.

Social Security Options

Over the years, numerous ideas have emerged about how to slow the future growth of Social Security. Generally, they fall into two categories: (1) slowing the rise in the level of initial benefits that people receive upon enrollment in the program, and (2) modifying or limiting the amount of cost-of-living adjustments (COLAs) they receive periodically after they are enrolled.

1. Slowing the growth of initial (or starting) benefits

The two most prominent ideas to slow the rise in initial benefits are (a) raising the age for receipt of full retirement benefits and (b) changing the benefit computation rules so that the initial benefits for each newly eligible age group rise as "prices" in the economy rise, rather than as average "wages" rise. It should be understood that, while these two ideas involve different approaches, they both limit the program's growth and can be structured to produce roughly the same degree of long-range savings. There are a few differences that are elaborated on below.

Raising the age for full benefits
This year, the age at which full retirement benefits can be paid to a newly eligible recipient is 66. Reduced retirement benefits can begin as early as age 62. As a general rule, early or late retirement will give you about the same total Social Security benefits over your lifetime. If you retire early, the monthly amounts will be smaller, to take into account the longer period over which you will receive them. If you retire late, you will get benefits for a shorter period of time, but the monthly amounts will be larger to make up for the time when you received nothing. Beginning with those people newly eligible in 2017 (defined as someone who reaches age 62 in that year), the full-benefit age will rise by two months a year until it reaches 67 for those newly eligible in 2022 and thereafter.

One spending-constraint option frequently mentioned is to allow the full-benefit age to rise gradually to 70. The measure would still allow reduced benefits at age 62, but the amount of reduction would be increased.

Converting to a system of "price indexing"
Each year, the Social Security benefit formula is modified to reflect the amount that average wages may have risen in the economy, creating a new and more generous formula for each newly eligible group of recipients. This annual updating is referred to as "wage indexing." By adjusting the formula in this manner, the amount that Social Security represents at the time of initial enrollment as a percentage of one's

former earnings from work stays roughly the same from one generation to the next—creating what are called "constant replacement rates." As the full-benefit age rises over the next several years—to 67 in 2022—there will be a reduction in those rates, for this period only, after which replacement rates will become constant again once the full-benefit age reaches 67.

Under an alternative procedure referred to as "price indexing," the annual adjustment to the benefit formula would be based on inflation (increases in prices) rather than wages. Since prices tend to rise more slowly than wages, the starting benefits of each newly eligible group of recipients would not be expected to rise as much as under current law.

2. Constraining Social Security COLAs

Once a person becomes eligible for Social Security, his or her benefits are increased periodically if the cost of living rises—typically annually. A COLA is triggered if the cost of living rises from the third quarter of the last year in which a COLA was provided to the third quarter of the current year (measured by the Bureau of Labor Statistics' Consumer Price Index for Wage Earners and Salaried Workers, or CPI-W). If the CPI-W rises by 0.1 percent or more, a COLA becomes payable the following January. If it doesn't rise, no COLA is provided, as was the case in 2010 and 2011 (the CPI-W actually declined over the first measuring period).

One option thought to produce savings would alter COLAs to reduce the overstatement of inflation embedded in the current CPI-W measurement. This would involve using a so-called "chained" CPI in lieu of the CPI-W (the chained measure would take into account consumers' propensity to buy other products or brands when the prices of their usual purchases rise). A second, stronger approach would be to make COLAs equal to the increase in the CPI minus one percentage point. A third would provide a COLA every two years unless inflation exceeded 5 percent in a one-year measuring period.

Appendix

Across-the-Board Spending and Revenue Options

Indexing of the income-tax brackets for inflation—which keeps people's incomes from edging into higher brackets—constrains revenues. Automatic hikes of the standard deduction and personal exemptions do too. COLAs in Social Security and other entitlement programs cause spending to rise from year to year. Automatic adjustments in Medicare fee schedules for hospitals and doctors keep health-care expenditures growing at a rapid clip. Thresholds for eligibility and payments under various means-tested and other support programs are automatically raised to keep "eligible" people enrolled and allow higher reimbursements.

A number of approaches for constraining indexing and related across-the-board measures are listed below:

1. Require the use of a chained CPI for all indexing provisions that tie revenues or spending to the cost of living;
2. Reduce all cost-of-living adjustments in spending programs by one percentage point (except anti-poverty programs);
3. Reduce all forms of annual spending and revenue cost-of-living adjustments by one percentage point;
4. Suspend all forms of annual spending and revenue cost-of-living adjustments for a period of time—perhaps three to five years— or permanently make the adjustments biennial instead of annual;
5. Place limits on the growth of all categories of discretionary spending.

Brief Descriptions of Medicare, Medicaid, Social Security, and "All-Other" Spending

Medicare

Medicare is a federal health-insurance program for persons aged 65 and older as well as for some individuals with disabilities. It covers nearly 50 million Americans, and the program is expected to spend $570 billion in 2012.

The traditional Medicare program pays benefits on a fee-for-service basis. About 35 million recipients are enrolled in traditional Medicare. As an alternative, recipients may enroll in private health plans under the Medicare Advantage program instead of traditional Medicare. An estimated 13 million recipients will participate in these plans in 2012. Medicare Advantage plans cover the same basic services as traditional Medicare, and they may offer additional benefits or lower costs to enrollees. Those plans are paid a monthly amount per enrollee to cover the cost of their care.

Medicare has four components: Hospital Insurance (Part A), Supplementary Medical Insurance (Part B), Medicare Advantage Program (Part C), and Prescription-Drug Coverage (Part D).

Medicare Hospital Insurance, Part A

Medicare Part A helps pay for hospital, home-health, nursing-facility, and hospice care. It is largely funded by taxing 2.9 percent of a worker's total annual earnings[1] (half paid by the employee and half by the employer). Individuals are entitled to coverage under Part A if they have a sufficient period of employment. Recipients are subject to cost-sharing requirements, including an initial deductible for hospitalization (equal to the cost of the first day of care, or $1,156 in 2012) and coinsurance for long hospital stays or the use of nursing-home care.

Medicare Supplementary Medical Insurance, Part B

Medicare Part B covers physician, outpatient, home-health care, and preventive services. It is funded through recipient premiums (covering 25 percent of program costs) and the Treasury's general revenues (primarily the income tax and public borrowing, which cover the remaining costs). Although Part B is voluntary, most eligible individuals enroll in the program. The monthly premium in 2012 is $99.90 for individuals who have annual incomes up to $85,000 (or double that for a couple), with higher-income recipients paying a higher premium. Recipients are subject to an annual deductible ($140 in 2012) and pay 20 percent of Medicare-approved charges for their care.

Because traditional Medicare requires out-of-pocket expenditures (such as deductibles and coinsurance), many recipients also have supplemental coverage. This may be purchased in the private insurance market, supplied through retiree health insurance, or, for low-income individuals, provided through Medicaid.

---

1. This is in contrast to Social Security payroll taxation where the tax is levied on earnings up to an annual cap, which this year is set at $110,100.

Medicare Advantage Program, Part C

Medicare Advantage offers a private-plan alternative to the traditional Medicare system. Recipients can enroll in comprehensive, competing private health plans, including health-maintenance organizations (HMOs), preferred-provider organizations (PPOs), and private fee-for-service plans. These plans cover all Part A and Part B services, and they generally offer a prescription-drug benefit under Part D. Medicare pays the plans based on a bidding system; as of 2007, all Advantage plan payments are adjusted to reflect the health-risk profiles of their enrollees.

Medicare Prescription-Drug Coverage, Part D

Medicare Part D is an optional outpatient prescription-drug benefit, distributed through private plans. Like Part B, 25 percent of the cost of Part D is funded through beneficiary premiums and the remaining cost is paid through general tax revenues or public borrowing. Unlike Part B, Medicare's payments to individual plans and for enrollee premiums are based on a competitive bidding process. The average monthly premium is estimated to be $38 in 2012. In addition to the monthly premium, higher-income enrollees (households with income exceeding $170,000 or individuals with income greater than $85,000) will pay between $11.60 and $66.40 per month. Part D plans are allowed to vary their benefits and coverage of specific drugs so long as the actuarial value of the benefit equals that of a standard plan. Many plans do not require an annual deductible, but all plans require that enrollees pay either a fixed-dollar copayment or coinsurance (which varies with the cost of the drug).

Medicaid

Medicaid is a shared federal-state entitlement program for low-income people. It was enacted, along with Medicare, in 1965. The program is operated by the states, with each state receiving federal matching funds for the costs it incurs in paying health-care providers for their services to enrollees. To be eligible, enrollees must have incomes and resources below certain levels, which vary from state to state. States are not required to participate in the program, but since 1982, all 50 states have chosen to do so.

The program's benefits cover basic health-care and long-term-care services, with about 60 percent going toward hospital and other acute-care services, and the remainder paying for nursing-home and long-term care.

While state participation is voluntary, certain basic services must be provided, including hospital care (both inpatient and outpatient), nursing-home care, physician services, laboratory and diagnostic X-ray services, immunizations and other screening, diagnostic and treat-ment services for children, family planning, health-center and rural health-clinic services, nurse-midwife and nurse-practitioner services, and physician-assistant services.

Because states are allowed to design their own benefits packages as long as they meet the minimum federal requirements, Medicaid benefits vary considerably from state to state. About half of all Medicaid spend-ing covers groups of people and services above the federal minimum.

In 2012, the program is estimated to cover 68 million low-income people. Children are the largest group, numbering 33 million. Low-income non-aged adults will number 29 million, 11 million of whom are blind and disabled. And seniors, aged 65 and older, will number 6 million. The significance of the latter group is reflected by Medicaid's status as the nation's largest single purchaser of long-term and nursing-home care.

The program is by far the government's most expensive general-welfare program. The federal government covers about 57 percent of the costs, and the states pay for the remaining 43 percent.[2] While

---

2. On average from FY 2012 to FY 2013, federal Medicaid payments will represent approximately 57 percent of total Medicaid spending. The 2010 health-care legislation,

nearly half of Medicaid's enrollees are children, the majority of the federal money (65 percent) goes for services for the elderly and disabled. In 2012, average per-person spending on the aged is estimated to be $11,340; the average for a child is estimated to be $1,550. The single largest portion of Medicaid money pays for long-term care for the elderly. A little more than 20 percent of the federal Medicaid share is spent on services for children.

Social Security

Social Security is the federal government's largest nondefense program. Created in 1935, the program now consists of two parts: Old-Age and Survivors Insurance (OASI), which pays benefits to retired workers and to their dependents and survivors, and Disability Insurance (DI), which makes payments to disabled workers and to their dependents. In all, nearly 57 million people are receiving Social Security benefits. CBO projects expenditures of $760 billion in fiscal year 2012, or roughly one-fifth of the federal budget.

In general, workers are eligible for retirement benefits if they are 62 or older and have paid sufficient Social Security taxes for at least 10 years. Workers whose employment has been limited because of a physical or mental disability can become eligible for DI benefits at an earlier age and, in many cases, with a shorter employment history. Various rules for determining eligibility and benefit amounts apply to family members of retired, disabled, or deceased workers.

When retired or disabled workers first claim Social Security benefits, the initial payments they receive are based on their average lifetime earnings. The formula used to translate average earnings into

---

which among its many provisions expands Medicaid coverage starting in 2014, will provide enhanced federal matching rates for certain eligible populations, leading to an average federal share for Medicaid that ranges between 60 percent and 62 percent, depending on the year.

benefits is progressive; that is, it replaces a larger share of preretirement earnings for people with lower average earnings than it does for people with higher earnings. The benefit formula and individual earnings histories are indexed to changes in average annual earnings for the labor force as a whole. Because average national earnings generally grow at a faster rate than inflation, that indexation causes initial benefits for future recipients to grow in real (inflation-adjusted) terms—meaning they can buy more.

For retirement benefits, a final adjustment is made on the basis of the age at which a recipient chooses to start claiming benefits: the longer a person waits (up to age 70), the higher the benefits will be. That final adjustment is intended to be "actuarially fair," so that an individual's total lifetime benefits will have an approximately equal value regardless of when he or she begins collecting them.

Once a person joins the rolls, his or her subsequent benefits are raised through COLAs (typically once a year) to reflect increases in consumer prices, depending if and how high prices rise.

For workers born before 1938, the age of eligibility for full retirement benefits—referred to as Social Security's normal retirement age—is 65. Under current law, that age is gradually increasing and will be 67 for people born in 1960 or later. Specifically, the normal retirement age rose by two months per birth year for people born between 1938 and 1943, remains at 66 for those born between 1944 and 1954, and then begins to increase again by two months per birth year for people born between 1955 and 1960. The age at which workers may start receiving reduced benefits—62—remains the same.

About 64 percent of recipients receive their payments as retired workers, 15 percent as disabled workers, 13 percent as survivors of deceased workers, and the remaining 9 percent as spouses or children of retired or disabled workers.

The program has two sources of tax revenues. The main one is a tax on 12.4 percent of earnings, split evenly by workers and their employers. Only earnings up to a maximum annual amount ($110,100 in 2012) are subject to the payroll tax. That amount—the taxable-earnings base—is adjusted each year for changes in average earnings unless the cost-of-living adjustment is zero, in which case it remains unchanged. The other, smaller source, which is equal to about 3 percent of tax revenues, is the income taxes that higher-income recipients pay on their benefits.

The "All-Other" Category of the Budget

There are three basic components of "all-other" spending:

Discretionary
1. Defense spending.
2. Domestic and international spending.

Mandatory
3. Spending for entitlement programs other than Medicare, Medicaid, and Social Security.

This is the largest and most diverse category of the federal budget. Today, it accounts for 57 percent of overall federal spending other than for interest on the debt. However, to label it as a category is a bit of an oversimplification, as it is the amalgamation of a vast number of federal programs and spending activities. The discretionary portion consists of hundreds of programs and categories of government activity for which Congress typically appropriates spending. The mandatory portion consists of entitlement programs such as unemployment insurance, public-assistance programs (e.g., SSI, TANF, and food stamps), federal civil-service-retirement programs, and veterans' service-related compensation and pensions, among others. This latter category differs from discretionary programs in that its spending is largely set for lengthy or indefinite periods by the laws that created each of them, not by annual appropriations.

The discretionary side, other than defense, includes NIH research, the promotion of science and technology, energy development and assistance, homeland security, veteran's health services, education programs, housing programs, agricultural support, transportation, the national parks, NASA, environmental protection, and a host of other local and national activities.

Spending in this all-other category, taken as a whole, is larger today than the spending made under the big three entitlement programs, but it is not projected to remain so, as the nation's aging baby boomers increasingly drive up spending for Medicare, Medicaid, and Social Security. Generally, most analysts who have studied the federal budget see the all-other category as an area where spending as a share of the economy will subside in the years to come. The general trend line over the past 50 years has been downward, dropping steadily from a level of close to 15 percent of the economy in the 1960s to anywhere from 8 percent to 10 percent, until a recent spike caused by war spending and recession relief.

Defense spending dropped from 9.3 percent of the economy in 1960s to 3 percent at the turn of the century, and even with the nation engaged in two recent wars, it rose only to 4.8 percent in 2010. The domestic side peaked decades ago as well, reaching a high of 9.1 percent in 1976. The discretionary portion of the domestic side—accounting for more than of half of that spending—reached a high of 5.2 percent in 1980, and for most of the last three decades it has hovered in the mid–3 percent range. In the last three years it spiked up again—largely due to spending to dampen the recession's affects—but with recently enacted caps, CBO projects, it will drop significantly over the next decade.

Nonetheless, taken as whole, this broad category of spending is projected to account for a substantial portion of future federal spending—ranging from 11.5 percent of the economy today to 8 percent to 10 percent in the long run. When looking for budget savings, it is hard to ignore something as large as one-tenth of the economy, even if that consumption does not contribute to the spiraling fiscal trend line. That said, given the multitude of discretionary programs, it also may be the hardest to rein in politically, in that constraining it will bring out many difficult disputes by the vast number of interests affected.

While an approach that attempts to prioritize spending among those interests may be difficult, broad-scale or across-the-board constraints have been enacted at various times, most recently last year, when spending caps were put in place and future spending-reduction triggers were put into effect encompassing large components of discretionary spending that could impose further constraints on both defense and domestic appropriations.

ABOUT THE AUTHOR

DAVID KOITZ spent 25 years as a policy analyst on Capitol Hill. Following his early years detailed to Congressman Jake Pickle's Social Security Subcommittee in the House of Representatives, he spent more than two decades working with many members of Congress as a legislative specialist at the Congressional Research Service of the Library of Congress, and later as a senior staff advisor at the Congressional Budget Office. He was well known as a seasoned source for independent advice on legislation affecting federal entitlements and the budget generally. He worked regularly with the House Ways and Means and Senate Finance Committees, with the Budget and Aging Committees of both chambers, testifying on numerous occasions and often preparing reports for committees and their chairmen about programs under their jurisdiction. His reports and policy briefs number in the hundreds. He gave counsel to various members of Greenspan Social Security Commission in 1983, to the Bipartisan Entitlement Commission in 1995, to numerous independent panels and commissions examining federal entitlements, pensions, health care, disability insurance, the administration of social security, the Social Security and Medicare trustees' reports, and to various caucuses and congressional factions of both houses and both parties.

In the years since leaving the Hill, he served as a policy consultant to Senator Gordon Smith during his tenure as chairman of the Senate Aging Committee and as a member of the Senate Finance Committee.

Among his other clients were the White House Conference on Aging, the Concord Coalition, the Heinz Family Foundation, the Committee for a Responsible Federal Budget, the Department of Health and Human Services, and the Social Security Administration. He received distinguished service awards from the Department of Health, Education, and Welfare, the Congressional Research Service, and the National Academy of Social Insurance for his work with Congress. This monograph is his second publication for the Hoover Institution—the first, *Seeking Middle Ground on Social Security Reform,* published in 2001, sought to disentangle the complex politics of both political parties as they pursued their respective reforms of Social Security. He and his wife continue to reside in the Washington, D.C. area.

INDEX